Virtual Clinical Excursions—Pediatrics

for

Wong's Nursing Care of Infants and Children
9th Edition

prepared by

David Wilson, MS, RNC
Adjunct Faculty
Langston University School of Nursing

Staff Nurse
Children's Hospital Urgent Care Center
Saint Francis Hospital
Tulsa, Oklahoma

Marilyn J. Hockenberry, PhD, RN-CS, PNP, FAAN
Director, Center for Clinical Research and
Evidence-Based Practice
Nurse Scientist, Texas Children's Hospital

Director of Nurse Practitioners
Texas Children's Cancer Center

Professor, Department of Pedia   s
Baylor College of Medicine
Houston, Texas

Patrick B
Assist
Evidenc
                    ..as

software developed by

Wolfsong Informatics, LLC
Tucson, Arizona

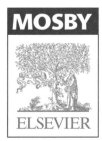

3251 Riverport Lane
Maryland Heights, Missouri 63043

VIRTUAL CLINICAL EXCURSIONS—PEDIATRICS FOR
WONG'S NURSING CARE OF INFANTS AND CHILDREN,
NINTH EDITION
Copyright © 2011, 2007 by Mosby, Inc., an affiliate of Elsevier Inc.

ISBN: 978-0-323-07972-3

Notice

Knowledge and best practice in this field are constantly changing. As new research and experience broaden our knowledge, changes in practice, treatment and drug therapy may become necessary or appropriate. Readers are advised to check the most current information provided (i) on procedures featured or (ii) by the manufacturer of each product to be administered, to verify the recommended dose or formula, the method and duration of administration, and contraindications. It is the responsibility of the practitioner, relying on their own experience and knowledge of the patient, to make diagnoses, to determine dosages and the best treatment for each individual patient, and to take all appropriate safety precautions. To the fullest extent of the law, neither the Publisher nor the Authors assumes any liability for any injury and/or damage to persons or property arising out or related to any use of the material contained in this book.

ISBN: 978-0-323-07972-3

Vice President and Publisher: *Tom Wilhelm*
Editor: *Jeff Downing*
Associate Developmental Editor: *Krissy Prysmiki*
Publishing Services Manager: *Jeff Patterson*
Project Manager: *Tracey Schriefer*

Printed in the United States of America

Last digit is the print number: 9   8   7   6   5   4   3   2   1

Workbook
prepared by

David Wilson, MS, RNC
Adjunct Faculty
Langston University School of Nursing

Staff Nurse
Children's Hospital Urgent Care Center
Saint Francis Hospital
Tulsa, Oklahoma

Marilyn J. Hockenberry, PhD, RN-CS, PNP, FAAN
Director, Center for Clinical Research and
Evidence-Based Practice
Nurse Scientist, Texas Children's Hospital

Director of Nurse Practitioners
Texas Children's Cancer Center

Professor, Department of Pediatrics
Baylor College of Medicine
Houston, Texas

Contributing Editor

Patrick Barrera, BS
Research Program Coordinator
Center for Nursing Research
Texas Children's Hospital
Houston, Texas

Textbook

Marilyn J. Hockenberry, PhD, RN-CS, PNP, FAAN
Director, Center for Clinical Research and Evidence-Based Practice
Nurse Scientist, Texas Children's Hospital

Director of Nurse Practitioners
Texas Children's Cancer Center

Professor, Department of Pediatrics
Baylor College of Medicine
Houston, Texas

David Wilson, MS, RNC
Adjunct Faculty
Langston University School of Nursing

Staff Nurse
Children's Hospital Urgent Care Center
Saint Francis Hospital
Tulsa, Oklahoma

Reviewers

Gina Long, RN, DNSc
Assistant Professor
Department of Nursing
College of Health Professions
Northern Arizona University
Flagstaff, Arizona

Diana Mixon
Associate Professor
Department of Nursing
Boise State University
Boise, Idaho

Contents

Table of Contents
Wong's Nursing Care of Infants and Children, 9th Edition

Getting Started

GETTING SET UP

■ MINIMUM SYSTEM REQUIREMENTS

WINDOWS®

Windows Vista®, XP, 2000 (Recommend Windows XP/2000)
Pentium® III processor (or equivalent) @ 600 MHz (Recommend 800 MHz or better)
256 MB of RAM (Recommend 1 GB or more for Windows Vista)
800 x 600 screen size (Recommend 1024 x 768)
Thousands of colors
12x CD-ROM drive

Note: Windows Vista and XP require administrator privileges for installation.

MACINTOSH®

MAC OS X (up to 10.6.1)
Apple Power PC G3 @ 500 MHz or better
128 MB of RAM (Recommend 256 MB or more)
800 x 600 screen size (Recommend 1024 x 768)
Thousands of colors
12x CD-ROM drive
Stereo speakers or headphones

■ INSTALLATION INSTRUCTIONS

WINDOWS

1. Insert the *Virtual Clinical Excursions—Pediatrics* CD-ROM.
2. The setup screen should appear automatically if the current product is not already installed. Windows Vista users may be asked to authorize additional security prompts.
3. Follow the onscreen instructions during the setup process.

   If the setup screen does *not* appear automatically (and *Virtual Clinical Excursions—Pediatrics* has not been installed already):
   a. Click the **My Computer** icon on your desktop or on your Start menu.
   b. Double-click on your CD-ROM drive.
   c. If installation does not start at this point:
      (1) Click the **Start** icon on the taskbar and select the **Run** option.
      (2) Type d:\setup.exe (where "d:\" is your CD-ROM drive) and press **OK**.
      (3) Follow the onscreen instructions for installation.

MACINTOSH

1. Insert the *Virtual Clinical Excursions—Pediatrics* CD in the CD-ROM drive. The disk icon will appear on your desktop.

2. Double-click on the disk icon.

3. Double-click on the VCEPE_MAC run file.

Note: Virtual Clinical Excursions—Pediatrics for Macintosh does not have an installation setup and can only be run directly from the CD.

■ HOW TO USE VIRTUAL CLINICAL EXCURSIONS—PEDIATRICS

WINDOWS

1. Double-click on the *Virtual Clinical Excursions—Pediatrics* icon located on your desktop.
2. Or navigate to the program via the Windows Start menu.

Note: If your computer uses Windows Vista, right-click on the desktop shortcut and choose **Properties**. In the Compatibility Mode, check the box for "Run as Administrator." Below is a screen capture to show what this looks like.

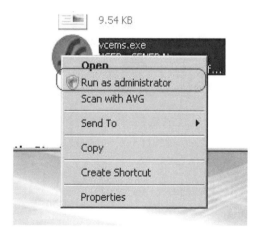

1. Insert the *Virtual Clinical Excursions—Pediatrics* CD in the CD-ROM drive. The disk icon will appear on your desktop.
2. Double-click on the disk icon.
3. Double-click on the VCEPE_MAC run file.

■ SCREEN SETTINGS

For best results, your computer monitor resolution should be set at a minimum of 800 x 600. The number of colors displayed should be set to "thousands or higher" (High Color or 16 bit) or "millions of colors" (True Color or 24 bit).

Windows

1. From the **Start** menu, select **Control Panel** (on some systems, you will first go to **Settings**, then to **Control Panel**).
2. Double-click on the **Display** icon.
3. Click on the **Settings** tab.
4. Under **Screen resolution** use the slider bar to select **800 by 600 pixels**.
5. Access the **Colors** drop-down menu by clicking on the down arrow.
6. Select **High Color (16 bit)** or **True Color (24 bit)**.
7. Click on **OK**.
8. You may be asked to verify the setting changes. Click **Yes**.
9. You may be asked to restart your computer to accept the changes. Click **Yes**.

Macintosh

1. Select the **Monitors** control panel.
2. Select **800 x 600** (or similar) from the **Resolution** area.
3. Select **Thousands** or **Millions** from the **Color Depth** area.

■ WEB BROWSERS

Supported web browsers include Microsoft Internet Explorer (IE) version 6.0 or higher, Netscape version 7.1 or higher, and Mozilla version 1.4 or higher.

If you use America Online® (AOL) for web access, you will need AOL version 4.0 or higher and one of the browsers listed above. Do not use earlier versions of AOL with earlier versions of IE, because you will have difficulty accessing many features.

For best results with AOL:
- Connect to the Internet using AOL version 4.0 or higher.
- Open a private chat within AOL (this allows the AOL client to remain open, without asking whether you wish to disconnect while minimized).
- Minimize AOL.
- Launch a recommended browser.

■ **TECHNICAL SUPPORT**

Technical support for this product is available 24 hours a day, seven days a week, excluding holidays. Before calling, be sure that your computer meets the minimum system requirements to run this software. Inside the United States and Canada, call 1-800-692-9010. Outside North America, call 314-447-8094. You may also fax your questions to 314-447-8078 or contact Technical Support through e-mail: technical.support@elsevier.com.

Trademarks: Windows, Macintosh, Pentium, and America Online are registered trademarks.

Copyright © 2011, 2007 by Mosby, Inc., an affiliate of Elsevier Inc.

All rights reserved. No part of this product may be reproduced or transmitted in any form or by any means, electronic or mechanical, including input or storage in any information system, without written permission from the publisher.

ACCESSING *Virtual Clinical Excursions—Pediatrics* FROM EVOLVE ⸻

The product you have purchased is part of the Evolve family of online courses and learning resources. Please read the following information thoroughly to get started.

To access your instructor's course on Evolve:

Your instructor will provide you with the username and password needed to access this specific course on the Evolve Learning System. Once you have received this information, please follow these instructions:

1. Go to the Evolve student page (http://evolve.elsevier.com/student).

2. Enter your username and password in the **Login to My Evolve** area and click the **Login** button.

3. You will be taken to your personalized **My Evolve** page, where the course will be listed in the **My Courses** module.

TECHNICAL REQUIREMENTS

To use an Evolve course, you will need access to a computer that is connected to the Internet and equipped with web browser software that supports frames. For optimal performance, it is recommended that you have speakers and use a high-speed Internet connection. However, slower dial-up modems (56 K minimum) are acceptable.

Whichever browser you use, the browser preferences must be set to enable cookies and the cache must be set to reload every time.

Enable Cookies

Browser	Steps
Internet Explorer (IE) 6.0 or higher	1. Select **Tools → Internet Options**. 2. Select **Privacy** tab. 3. Use the slider (slide down) to **Accept All Cookies**. 4. Click **OK**. -OR- 3. Click the **Advanced** button. 4. Click the check box next to **Override Automatic Cookie Handling**. 5. Click the **Accept** radio buttons under **First-party Cookies** and **Third-party Cookies**. 6. Click **OK**.
Mozilla Firefox 2.0 or higher	1. Select **Tools → Options**. 2. Select the **Privacy** icon. 3. Click to expand Cookies. 4. Select **Allow sites to set cookies**. 5. Click **OK**.

Set Cache to Always Reload a Page

Browser	Steps
Internet Explorer (IE) 6.0 or higher	1. Select **Tools → Internet Options**. 2. Select **General** tab. 3. Go to the **Temporary Internet Files** and click the **Settings** button. 4. Select the radio button for **Every visit to the page** and click **OK** when complete.
Mozilla Firefox 2.0 or higher	1. Select **Tools → Options**. 2. Select the **Privacy** icon. 3. Click to expand Cache. 4. Set the value to "**0**" in the **Use up to: __ MB of disk space for the cache** field. 5. Click **OK**.

Plug-Ins

Adobe Acrobat Reader—With the free Acrobat Reader software, you can view and print Adobe PDF files. Many Evolve products offer student and instructor manuals, checklists, and more in this format!

Download at: http://www.adobe.com

Apple QuickTime—Install this to hear word pronunciations, heart and lung sounds, and many other helpful audio clips within Evolve Online Courses!

Download at: http://www.apple.com

Adobe Flash Player—This player will enhance your viewing of many Evolve web pages, as well as educational short-form to long-form animation within the Evolve Learning System!

Download at: http://www.adobe.com

Adobe Shockwave Player—Shockwave is best for viewing the many interactive learning activities within Evolve Online Courses!

Download at: http://www.adobe.com

Microsoft Word Viewer—With this viewer, Microsoft Word users can share documents with those who don't have Word, and users without Word can open and view Word documents. Many Evolve products have testbank, student and instructor manuals, and other documents available for downloading and viewing on your own computer!

Download at: http://www.microsoft.com

Microsoft PowerPoint Viewer—With this viewer, you can access PowerPoint 97, 2000, and 2002 presentations even if you don't have PowerPoint. Many Evolve products have slides available for downloading and viewing on your own computer!

Download at: http://www.microsoft.com

SUPPORT INFORMATION

Live phone support is available to customers in the United States and Canada at **800-401-9962** 24 hours a day, seven days a week. Support is also available through email at <u>evolve-support@ elsevier.com</u>.

Online 24/7 support can be accessed on the Evolve website (<u>http://evolve.elsevier.com</u>). Resources include:

- Guided tours
- Tutorials
- Frequently asked questions (FAQs)
- Online copies of course user guides
- And much more!

A QUICK TOUR

Welcome to *Virtual Clinical Excursions—Pediatrics*, a virtual hospital setting in which you can work with multiple complex patient simulations and also learn to access and evaluate the information resources that are essential for high-quality patient care. The virtual hospital, Pacific View Regional Hospital, has realistic architecture and access to patient rooms, a Nurses' Station, and a Medication Room.

■ BEFORE YOU START

Make sure you have your textbook nearby when you use the *Virtual Clinical Excursions—Pediatrics* CD. You will want to consult topic areas in your textbook frequently while working with the CD and using this workbook.

■ HOW TO SIGN IN

- Enter your name on the Student Nurse identification badge.
- Now choose one of the four periods of care in which to work. In Periods of Care 1 through 3, you can actively engage in patient assessment, entry of data in the electronic patient record (EPR), and medication administration. Period of Care 4 presents the day in review. Highlight and click the appropriate period of care. (For this quick tour, choose **Period of Care 1: 0730-0815**.)
- This takes you to the Patient List screen (see example on page 11). Only the patients on the Pediatrics Floor are available. Note that the virtual time is provided in the box at the lower left corner of the screen (0730, since we chose Period of Care 1).

Note: If you choose to work during Period of Care 4: 1900-2000, the Patient List screen is skipped since you are not able to visit patients or administer medications during the shift. Instead, you are taken directly to the Nurses' Station, where the records of all the patients on the floor are available for your review.

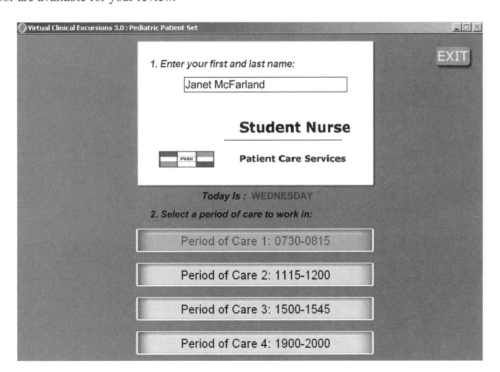

■ PATIENT LIST

PEDIATRICS UNIT

George Gonzalez (Room 301)
Diabetic ketoacidosis—An 11-year-old Hispanic male admitted for stabilization of blood glucose level and diabetic re-education associated with his diagnosis of type 1 diabetes mellitus. This patient's poor compliance with insulin therapy and dietary regime have resulted in frequent and repeated hospital admissions for diabetic ketoacidosis.

Tommy Douglas (Room 302)
Traumatic brain injury—A 6-year-old Caucasian male transferred from the Pediatric Intensive Care Unit in preparation for organ donation. This patient is status post ventriculostomy with negative intracerebral blood flow and requires extensive hemodynamic monitoring and support, along with compassionate family care.

Carrie Richards (Room 303)
Bronchiolitis—A 3½-month-old African-American female admitted with respiratory distress due to respiratory syncytial virus, along with dehydration and a poor nutritional status. Parent education and support are among her primary needs.

Stephanie Brown (Room 304)
Meningitis—A 3-year-old African-American female with a history of spastic cerebral palsy admitted for intravenous antibiotic therapy, neurologic monitoring, and support for a diagnosis of acute meningitis. Maintenance of physical and occupational programs addressing her mobility limitations complicate her acute care stay.

Tiffany Sheldon (Room 305)
Anorexia nervosa—A 14-year-old Caucasian female admitted for dehydration, electrolyte imbalance, and malnutrition following a syncope episode at home. This patient has a history of eating disorders, which have resulted in multiple hospital admissions and strained family dynamics between mother and daughter.

■ HOW TO SELECT A PATIENT

- You can choose one or more patients to work with from the Patient List by checking the box to the left of the patient name(s). For this quick tour, select Stephanie Brown. (In order to receive a scorecard for a patient, the patient must be selected before proceeding to the Nurses' Station.)
- Click on **Get Report** to the right of the medical records number (MRN) to view a summary of the patient's care during the 12-hour period before your arrival on the unit.
- After reviewing the report, click on **Go to Nurses' Station** in the right lower corner to begin your care. (*Note:* If you have been assigned to care for multiple patients, you can click on **Return to Patient List** to select and review the report for each additional patient before going to the Nurses' Station.)

Note: Even though the Patient List is initially skipped when you sign in to work for Period of Care 4, you can still access this screen if you wish to review the shift report for any of the patients. To do so, simply click on **Patient List** near the top left corner of the Nurses' Station (or click on the clipboard to the left of the Kardex). Then click on **Get Report** for the patient(s) whose care you are reviewing. This may be done during any period of care.

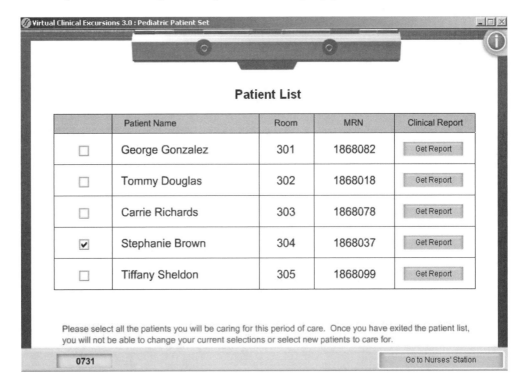

■ HOW TO FIND A PATIENT'S RECORDS

NURSES' STATION

Within the Nurses' Station, you will see:

1. A clipboard that contains the patient list for that floor.
2. A chart rack with patient charts labeled by room number, a notebook labeled Kardex, and a notebook labeled MAR (Medication Administration Record).
3. A desktop computer with access to the Electronic Patient Record (EPR).
4. A tool bar across the top of the screen that can also be used to access the Patient List, EPR, Chart, MAR, and Kardex. This tool bar is also accessible from each patient's room.
5. A Drug Guide containing information about the medications you are able to administer to your patients.
6. A tool bar across the bottom of the screen that can be used to access the Floor Map, patient rooms, Medication Room, and Drug Guide.

As you run your cursor over an item, it will be highlighted. To select, simply click on the item. As you use these resources, you will always be able to return to the Nurses' Station by clicking on the **Return to Nurses' Station** bar located in the right lower corner of your screen.

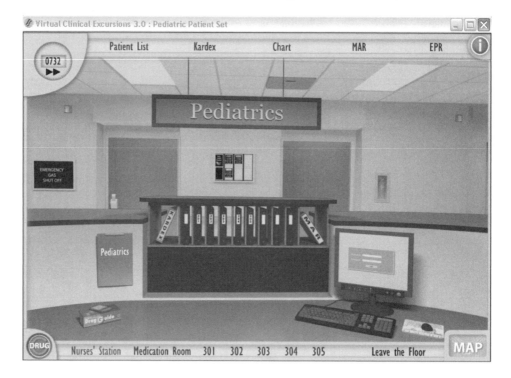

MEDICATION ADMINISTRATION RECORD (MAR)

The MAR icon located on the tool bar at the top of your screen accesses current 24-hour medications for each patient. Click on the icon and the MAR will open. (*Note:* You can also access the MAR by clicking on the MAR notebook on the far right side of the book rack in the center of the screen.) Within the MAR, tabs on the right side of the screen allow you to select patients by room number. Be careful to make sure you select the correct tab number for *your* patient rather than simply reading the first record that appears after the MAR opens. Each MAR sheet lists the following:

- Medications
- Route and dosage of each medication
- Times of administration of each medication

Note: The MAR changes each day. Expired MARs are stored in the patients' charts.

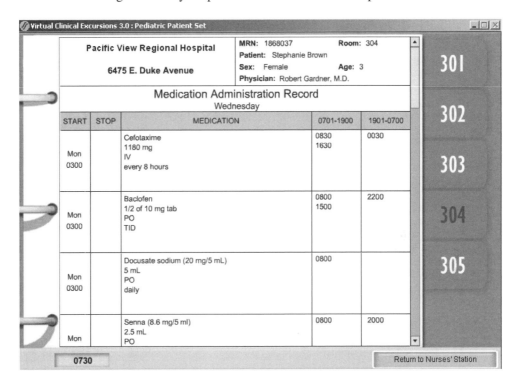

CHARTS

To access patient charts, either click on the **Chart** icon at the top of your screen or anywhere within the chart rack in the center of the Nurses' Station screen. When the close-up view appears, the individual charts are labeled by room number. To open a chart, click on the room number of the patient whose chart you wish to review. The patient's name and allergies will appear on the left side of the screen, along with a list of tabs on the right side of the screen, allowing you to view the following data:

- Allergies
- Physician's Orders
- Physician's Notes
- Nurse's Notes
- Laboratory Reports
- Diagnostic Reports
- Surgical Reports
- Consultations

- Patient Education
- History and Physical
- Nursing Admission
- Expired MARs
- Consents
- Mental Health
- Admissions
- Emergency Department

Information appears in real time. The entries are in reverse chronologic order, so use the down arrow at the right side of each chart page to scroll down to view previous entries. Flip from tab to tab to view multiple data fields or click on **Return to Nurses' Station** in the lower right corner of the screen to exit the chart.

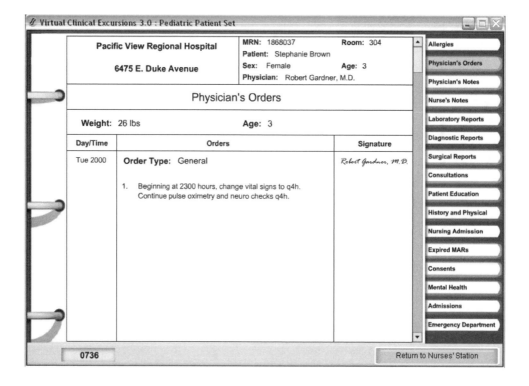

ELECTRONIC PATIENT RECORD (EPR)

The EPR can be accessed from the computer in the Nurses' Station or from the EPR icon located in the tool bar at the top of your screen. To access a patient's EPR:

- Click on either the computer screen or the **EPR** icon.
- Your username and password are automatically filled in.
- Click on **Login** to enter the EPR.
- *Note:* Like the MAR, the EPR is arranged numerically. Thus when you enter, you are initially shown the records of the patient in the lowest room number on the floor. To view the correct data for *your* patient, remember to select the correct room number, using the drop-down menu for the Patient field at the top left corner of the screen.

The EPR used in Pacific View Regional Hospital represents a composite of commercial versions being used in hospitals. You can access the EPR:

- to review existing data for a patient (by room number).
- to enter data you collect while working with a patient.

The EPR is updated daily, so no matter what day or part of a shift you are working, there will be a current EPR with the patient's data from the past days of the current hospital stay. This type of simulated EPR allows you to examine how data for different attributes have changed over time, as well as to examine data for all of a patient's attributes at a particular time. The EPR is fully functional (as it is in a real-life hospital). You can enter such data as blood pressure, breath sounds, and certain treatments. The EPR will not, however, allow you to enter data for a previous time period. Use the arrows at the bottom of the screen to move forward and backward in time.

Virtual Clinical Excursions 3.0 : Pediatric Patient Set

Patient: 304   Category: Vital Signs   **0731**

Name: Stephanie Brown	Tue 2300	Wed 0300	Wed 0700	Code Meanings	
PAIN: LOCATION				A	Abdomen
PAIN: RATING	0	0	0	Ar	Arm
PAIN: CHARACTERISTICS				B	Back
PAIN: VOCAL CUES				C	Chest
PAIN: FACIAL CUES				Ft	Foot
PAIN: BODILY CUES				H	Head
PAIN: SYSTEM CUES				Hd	Hand
PAIN: FUNCTIONAL EFFECTS				L	Left
PAIN: PREDISPOSING FACTORS				Lg	Leg
PAIN: RELIEVING FACTORS				Lw	Lower
PCA				N	Neck
TEMPERATURE (F)	98.6	98.6	97.6	NN	See Nurses notes
TEMPERATURE (C)				OS	Operative site
MODE OF MEASUREMENT	Ty	Ty	Ty	Or	See Physicians orders
SYSTOLIC PRESSURE	110	80	92	PN	See Progress notes
DIASTOLIC PRESSURE	60	42	50	R	Right
BP MODE OF MEASUREMENT	NIBP	NIBP	NIBP	Up	Upper
HEART RATE	82	98	92		
RESPIRATORY RATE	20	22	20		
SpO2 (%)	100	100	99		
BLOOD GLUCOSE					
WEIGHT			11.82		
HEIGHT					

Exit EPR

At the top of the EPR screen, you can choose patients by their room numbers. In addition, you have access to 17 different categories of patient data. To change patients or data categories, click the down arrow to the right of the room number or category.

The categories of patient data in the EPR are as follows:

- Vital Signs
- Respiratory
- Cardiovascular
- Neurologic
- Gastrointestinal
- Excretory
- Musculoskeletal
- Integumentary
- Reproductive
- Psychosocial
- Wounds and Drains
- Activity
- Hygiene and Comfort
- Safety
- Nutrition
- IV
- Intake and Output

Remember, each hospital selects its own codes. The codes used in the EPR at Pacific View Regional Hospital may be different from ones you have seen in your clinical rotations. Take some time to acquaint yourself with the codes. Within the Vital Signs category, click on any item in the left column (e.g., Pain: Characteristics). In the far-right column, you will see a list of code meanings for the possible findings and/or descriptors for that assessment area.

You will use the codes to record the data you collect as you work with patients. Click on the box in the last time column to the right of any item and wait for the code meanings applicable to that entry to appear. Select the appropriate code to describe your assessment findings and type it in the box. (*Note:* If no cursor appears within the box, click on the box again until the blue shading disappears and the blinking cursor appears.) Once the data are typed in this box, they are entered into the patient's record for this period of care only.

To leave the EPR, click on **Exit EPR** in the bottom right corner of the screen.

■ VISITING A PATIENT

From the Nurses' Station, click on the room number of the patient you wish to visit (in the tool bar at the bottom of your screen). Once you are inside the room, you will see a still photo of your patient in the top left corner. To verify that this is the correct patient, click on the **Check Armband** icon to the right of the photo. The patient's identification data will appear. If you click on **Check Allergies** (the next icon to the right), a list of the patient's allergies (if any) will replace the photo.

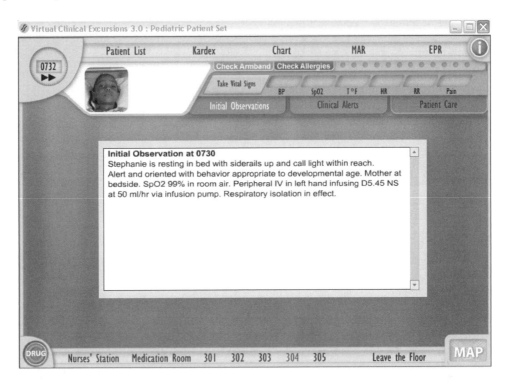

Also located in the patient's room are multiple icons you can use to assess the patient or the patient's medications. A virtual clock is provided in the upper left corner of the room to monitor your progress in real time. (*Note:* The fast-forward icon within the virtual clock will advance the time by 2-minute intervals when clicked.)

- The tool bar across the top of the screen allows you to check the **Patient List**, access the **EPR** to check or enter data, and view the patient's **Chart**, **MAR**, or **Kardex**.

- The **Take Vital Signs** icon allows you to measure the patient's up-to-the-minute blood pressure, oxygen saturation, temperature, heart rate, respiratory rate, and pain level.

- Each time you enter a patient's room, you are given an Initial Observation report to review (in the text box under the patient's photo). These notes are provided to give you a "look" at the patient as if you had just stepped into the room. You can also click on the **Initial Observations** icon to return to this box from other views within the patient's room. To the right of this icon is **Clinical Alerts**, a resource that allows you to make decisions about priority medication interventions based on emerging data collected in real time. Check this screen throughout your period of care to avoid missing critical information related to recently ordered or STAT medications.

- Clicking on **Patient Care** opens up three specific learning environments within the patient room: **Physical Assessment**, **Nurse-Client Interactions**, and **Medication Administration**.

- To perform a **Physical Assessment**, choose a body area (such as **Head & Neck**) from the column of yellow buttons. This activates a list of system subcategories for that body area (e.g., see **Sensory**, **Neurologic**, etc. in the green boxes). After you select the system you wish to evaluate, a brief description of the assessment findings will appear in a box to the right. A still photo provides a "snapshot" of how an assessment of this area might be done or what the finding might look like. For every body area, you can also click on **Equipment** on the right side of the screen.

- To the right of the Physical Assessment icon is **Nurse-Client Interactions**. Clicking on this icon will reveal the times and titles of any videos available for viewing. (*Note:* If the video you wish to see is not listed, this means you have not yet reached the correct virtual time to view that video. Check the virtual clock; you may return to access the video once its designated time has occurred—as long as you do so within the same period of care. Or you can click on the fast-forward icon within the virtual clock to advance the time by 2-minute intervals. You will then need to click again on **Patient Care** and **Nurse-Client Interactions** to refresh the screen.) To view a listed video, click on the white arrow to the right of the video title. Use the control buttons below the video to start, stop, pause, rewind, or fast-forward the action or to mute the sound.

- **Medication Administration** is the pathway that allows you to review and administer medications to a patient after you have prepared them in the Medication Room. This process is addressed further in the *How to Prepare Medications* section (pages 19-20) and in *Medications* (pages 26-30). For additional hands-on practice, see *Reducing Medication Errors* (pages 37-41).

■ HOW TO QUIT, CHANGE PATIENTS, OR CHANGE PERIODS OF CARE

How to Quit: From most screens, you may click the **Leave the Floor** icon on the bottom tool bar to the right of the patient room numbers. (*Note:* From some screens, you will first need to click an **Exit** button or **Return to Nurses' Station** before clicking **Leave the Floor**.) When the Floor Menu appears, click **Exit** to leave the program.

How to Change Patients or Periods of Care: To change patients, simply click on the new patient's room number. (You cannot receive a scorecard for a new patient, however, unless you have already selected that patient on the Patient List screen.) To change to a new period of care or to restart the virtual clock, click on **Leave the Floor** and then on **Restart the Program**.

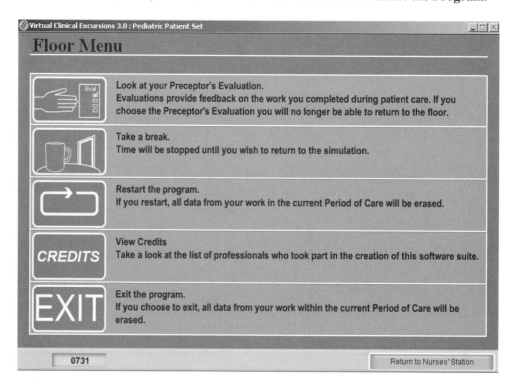

■ HOW TO PREPARE MEDICATIONS

From the Nurses' Station or the patient's room, you can access the Medication Room by clicking on the icon in the tool bar at the bottom of your screen to the left of the patient room numbers.

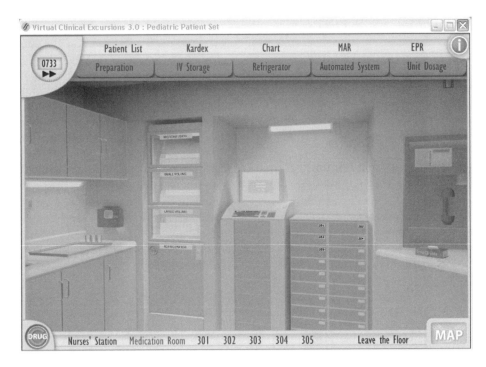

In the Medication Room you have access to the following (from left to right):

- A preparation area is located on the counter under the cabinets. To begin the medication preparation process, click on the tray on the counter or click on the **Preparation** icon at the top of the screen. The next screen leads you through a specific sequence (called the Preparation Wizard) to prepare medications one at a time for administration to a patient. However, no medication has been selected at this time. We will do this while working with a patient in *A Detailed Tour*. To exit this screen, click on **View Medication Room**.

- To the right of the cabinets (and above the refrigerator), IV storage bins are provided. Click on the bins themselves or on the **IV Storage** icon at the top of the screen. The bins are labeled **Microinfusion**, **Small Volume**, and **Large Volume**. Click on an individual bin to see a list of its contents. If you needed to prepare an IV medication at this time, you could click on the medication and its label would appear to the right under the patient's name. (*Note:* You can **Open** and **Close** any medication label by clicking the appropriate icon.) Next, you would click **Put Medication on Tray**. If you ever change your mind or decide that you have put the incorrect medication on the tray, you can reverse your actions by highlighting the medication on the tray and then clicking **Put Medication in Bin**. Click **Close Bin** in the right bottom corner to exit. **View Medication Room** brings you back to a full view of the entire room.

- A refrigerator is located under the IV storage bins to hold any medications that must be stored below room temperature. Click on the refrigerator door or on the **Refrigerator** icon at the top of the screen. Then click on the close-up view of the door to access the medications. When you are finished, click **Close Door** and then **View Medication Room**.

- To prepare controlled substances, click the **Automated System** icon at the top of the screen or click the computer monitor located to the right of the IV storage bins. A login screen will appear; your name and password are automatically filled in. Click **Login**. Select the patient for whom you wish to access medications; then select the correct medication drawer to open (they are stored alphabetically). Click **Open Drawer**, highlight the proper medication, and choose **Put Medication on Tray**. When you are finished, click **Close Drawer** and then **View Medication Room**.

- Next to the Automated System is a set of drawers identified by patient room number. To access these, click on the drawers or on the **Unit Dosage** icon at the top of the screen. This provides a close-up view of the drawers. To open a drawer, click on the room number of the patient you are working with. Next, click on the medication you would like to prepare for the patient, and a label will appear to the right, listing the medication strength, units, and dosage per unit. To exit, click **Close Drawer**; then click **View Medication Room**.

At any time, you can learn about a medication you wish to prepare for a patient by clicking on the **Drug** icon in the bottom left corner of the medication room screen or by clicking the **Drug Guide** book on the counter to the right of the unit dosage drawers. The **Drug Guide** provides information about the medications commonly included in nursing drug handbooks. Nutritional supplements and maintenance intravenous fluid preparations are not included. Highlight a medication in the alphabetical list; relevant information about the drug will appear in the screen below. To exit, click **Return to Medication Room**.

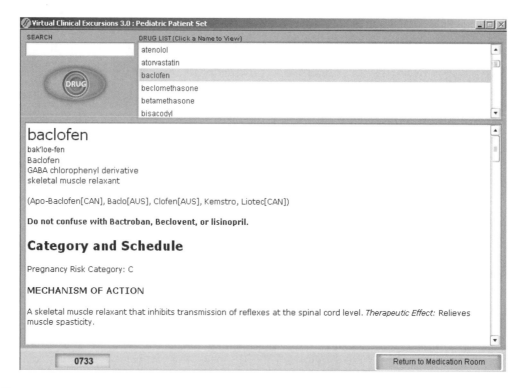

To access the MAR from the Medication Room and to review the medications ordered for a patient, click on the **MAR** icon located in the tool bar at the top of your screen and then click on the correct tab for your patient's room number. You may also click the **Review MAR** icon in the tool bar at the bottom of your screen from inside each medication storage area.

After you have chosen and prepared medications, go to the patient's room to administer them by clicking on the room number in the bottom tool bar. Inside the patient's room, click **Patient Care** and then **Medication Administration** and follow the proper administration sequence.

■ PRECEPTOR'S EVALUATIONS

When you have finished a session, click on **Leave the Floor** to go to the Floor Menu. At this point, you can click on the top icon (**Look at Your Preceptor's Evaluation**) to receive a scorecard that provides feedback on the work you completed during patient care.

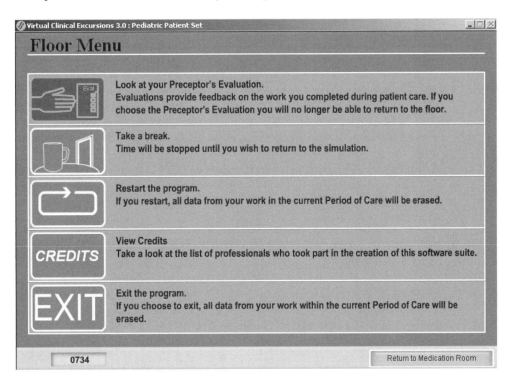

Evaluations are available for each patient you selected when you signed in for the current period of care. Click on the **Medication Scorecard** icon to see an example.

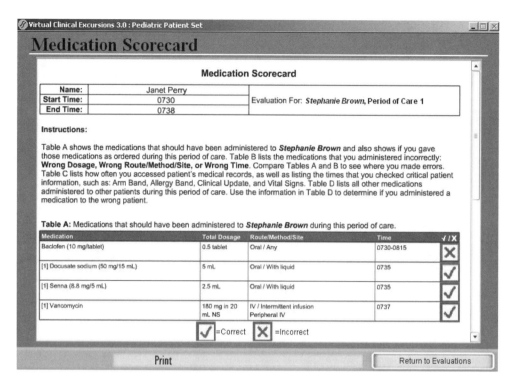

The scorecard compares the medications you administered to a patient during a period of care with what should have been administered. Table A lists the correct medications. Table B lists any medications that were administered incorrectly.

Remember, not every medication listed on the MAR should necessarily be given. For example, a patient might have an allergy to a drug that was ordered, or a medication might have been improperly transcribed to the MAR. Predetermined medication "errors" embedded within the program challenge you to exercise critical thinking skills and professional judgment when deciding to administer a medication, just as you would in a real hospital. Use all your available resources, such as the patient's chart and the MAR, to make your decision.

Table C lists the resources that were available to assist you in medication administration. It also documents whether and when you accessed these resources. For example, did you check the patient armband or perform a check of vital signs? If so, when?

You can click **Print** to get a copy of this report if needed. When you have finished reviewing the scorecard, click **Return to Evaluations** and then **Return to Menu**.

■ FLOOR MAP

To get a general sense of your location within the hospital, you can click on the **Map** icon found in the lower right corner of most of the screens in the *Virtual Clinical Excursions—Pediatrics* program. (*Note:* If you are following this quick tour step by step, you will need to **Restart the Program** from the Floor Menu, sign in again, and go to the Nurses' Station to access the map.) When you click the **Map** icon, a floor map appears, showing the layout of the floor you are currently on, as well as a directory of the patients and services on that floor. As you move your cursor over the directory list, the location of each room is highlighted on the map (and vice versa). The floor map can be accessed from the Nurses' Station, Medication Room, and each patient's room.

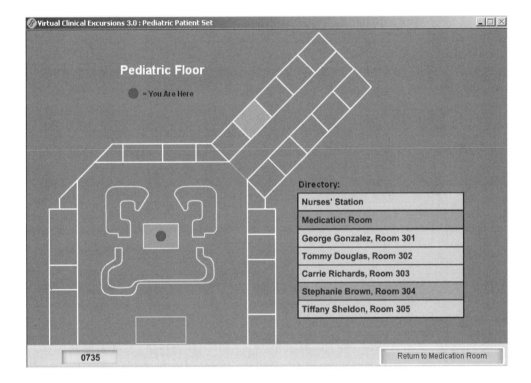

A DETAILED TOUR

If you wish to more thoroughly understand the capabilities of *Virtual Clinical Excursions—Pediatrics*, take a detailed tour by completing the following section. During this tour, we will work with a specific patient to introduce you to all the different components and learning opportunities available within the software.

■ WORKING WITH A PATIENT

Sign in for Period of Care 1 (0730-0815). From the Patient List, select Stephanie Brown in Room 304; however, do not go to the Nurses' Station yet.

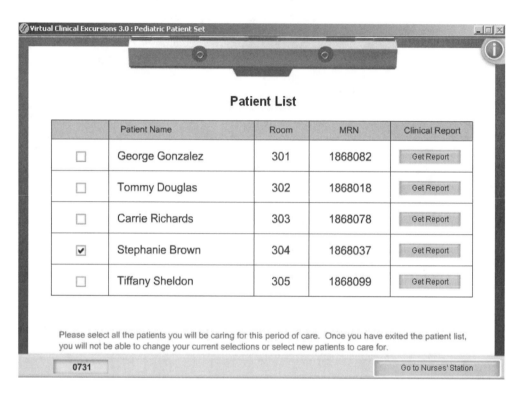

■ REPORT

In hospitals, when one shift ends and another begins, the outgoing nurse who attended a patient will give a verbal and sometimes a written summary of that patient's condition to the incoming nurse who will assume care for the patient. This summary is called a report and is an important source of data to provide an overview of a patient. Your first task is to get the clinical report on Stephanie Brown. To do this, click **Get Report** in the far right column in this patient's row. From a brief review of this summary, identify the problems and areas of concern that you will need to address for this patient.

When you have finished noting any areas of concern, click on **Go to Nurses' Station**.

■ CHARTS

You can access Stephanie Brown's chart from the Nurses' Station or from the patient's room (304). From the Nurses' Station, click on the chart rack or on the **Chart** icon in the tool bar at the top of your screen. Next, click on the chart labeled **304** to open the medical record for Stephanie Brown. Click on the **Emergency Department** tab to view a record of why this patient was admitted.

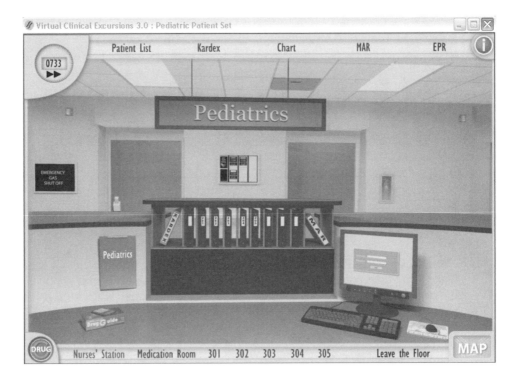

How many days has Stephanie Brown been in the hospital?

What tests were done upon her arrival in the Emergency Department and why?

What was her reason for admission?

You should also click on **Diagnostic Reports** to learn what additional tests or procedures were performed and when. Finally, review the **Nursing Admission** and **History and Physical** to learn about the health history of this patient. When you are done reviewing the chart, click **Return to Nurses' Station**.

■ MEDICATIONS

Open the Medication Administration Record (MAR) by clicking on the **MAR** icon in the tool bar at the top of your screen. *Remember:* The MAR automatically opens to the first occupied room number on the floor—which is not necessarily your patient's room number! Since you need to access Stephanie Brown's MAR, click on tab **304** (her room number). Always make sure you are giving the *Right Drug to the Right Patient!*

Examine the list of medications ordered for Stephanie Brown. In the table below, list the medications that need to be given during this period of care (0730-0815). For each medication, note the dosage, route, and time to be given.

Time	Medication	Dosage	Route

Click on **Return to Nurses' Station**. Next, click on **304** on the bottom tool bar and then verify that you are indeed in Stephanie Brown's room. Select **Clinical Alerts** (the icon to the right of Initial Observations) to check for any emerging data that might affect your medication administration priorities. Next, go to the patient's chart (click on the **Chart** icon; then click on **304**). When the chart opens, select the **Physician's Orders** tab.

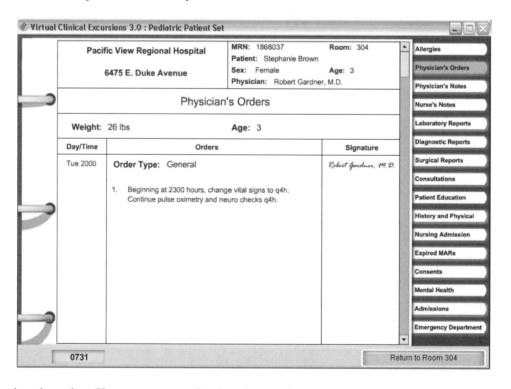

Review the orders. Have any new medications been ordered? Return to the MAR (click **Return to Room 304**; then click **MAR**). Verify that any new medications have been correctly transcribed to the MAR. Mistakes are sometimes made in the transcription process in the hospital setting, and it is sound practice to double-check any new order.

Are there any patient assessments you will need to perform before administering these medications? If so, return to Room 304 and click on **Patient Care** and then **Physical Assessment** to complete those assessments before proceeding.

Now click on the **Medication Room** icon in the tool bar at the bottom of your screen to locate and prepare the medications for Stephanie Brown.

In the Medication Room, you must access the medications for Stephanie Brown from the specific dispensing system in which each medication is stored. Locate each medication that needs to be given in this time period and click on **Put Medication on Tray** as appropriate. (*Hint:* Look in **Unit Dosage** drawer first.) When you are finished, click on **Close Drawer** and then on **View Medication Room**. Now click on the medication tray on the counter on the left side of the medication room screen to begin preparing the medications you have selected. (*Remember:* You can also click **Preparation** in the tool bar at top of the screen.)

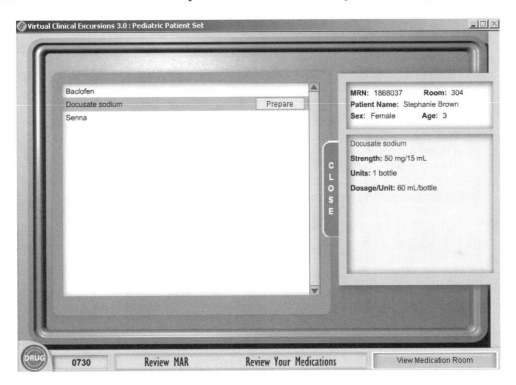

In the preparation area, you should see a list of the medications you put on the tray in the previous steps. Click on the first medication and then click **Prepare**. Follow the onscreen instructions of the Preparation Wizard, providing any data requested. As an example, let's follow the preparation process for docusate sodium, one of the medications due to be administered to Stephanie Brown during this period of care. To begin, click to select **Docusate sodium**; then click **Prepare**. Now work through the Preparation Wizard sequence as detailed below:

Amount of medication in the bottle: 60 mL.
Enter the amount of medication you will draw up into a syringe: **5** mL.
Click **Next**.
Select the patient you wish to set aside the medication for: **Room 304, Stephanie Brown**.
Click **Finish**.
Click **Return to Medication Room**.

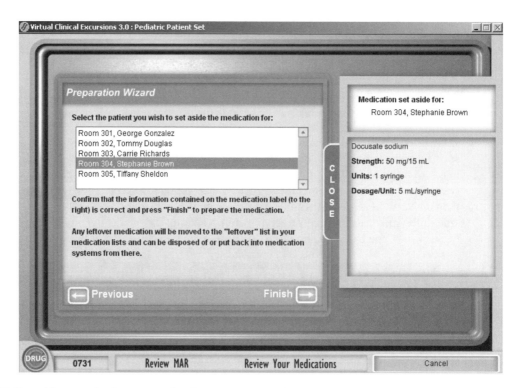

Follow this same basic process for the other medications due to be administered to Stephanie Brown during this period of care. (*Hint:* Look in **IV Storage** and **Automated System**.)

PREPARATION WIZARD EXCEPTIONS

- Some medications in *Virtual Clinical Excursions—Pediatrics* are preprepared by the pharmacy (e.g., IV antibiotics) and taken to the patient room as a whole. This is common practice in most hospitals.
- Blood products are not administered by students through the *Virtual Clinical Excursions—Pediatrics* simulations since blood administration follows specific protocols not covered in this program.
- The *Virtual Clinical Excursions—Pediatrics* simulations do not allow for mixing more than one type of medication, such as regular and Lente insulins, in the same syringe. In the clinical setting, when multiple types of insulin are ordered for a patient, the regular insulin is drawn up first, followed by the longer-acting insulin. Insulin is always administered in a special unit-marked syringe.

Now return to Room 304 (click on **304** on the bottom tool bar) to administer Stephanie Brown's medications.

At any time during the medication administration process, you can perform a further review of systems, take vital signs, check information contained within the chart, or verify patient identity and allergies. Inside Stephanie Brown's room, click **Take Vital Signs**. (*Note:* These findings change over time to reflect the temporal changes you would find in a patient similar to Stephanie Brown.)

When you have gathered all the data you need, click on **Patient Care** and then select **Medication Administration**. Any medications you prepared in the previous steps should be listed on the left side of your screen. Let's continue the administration process with the vancomycin ordered for Stephanie Brown. Click to highlight **Vancomycin** in the list of medications. Next, click on the down arrow to the right of **Select** and choose **Administer** from the drop-down menu. This will activate the Administration Wizard. Complete the Wizard sequence as follows:

- Route: **IV**
- Method: **Intermittent Infusion**
- Site: **Peripheral IV**
- Click **Administer to Patient** arrow.
- Would you like to document this administration in the MAR? **Yes**
- Click **Finish** arrow.

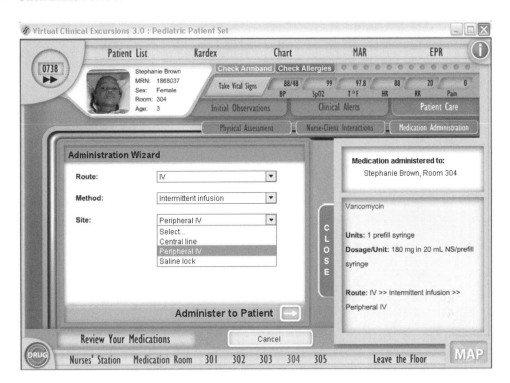

Your selections are recorded by a tracking system and evaluated on a Medication Scorecard stored under Preceptor's Evaluations. This scorecard can be viewed, printed, and given to your instructor. To access the Preceptor's Evaluations, click on **Leave the Floor**. When the Floor Menu appears, select **Look at Your Preceptor's Evaluation**. Then click on **Medication Scorecard** inside the box with Stephanie Brown's name (see example on the following page).

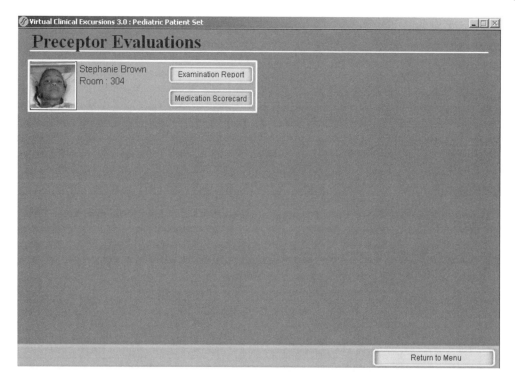

MEDICATION SCORECARD

- First, review Table A. Was vancomycin given correctly? Did you give the other medications as ordered?
- Table B shows you which (if any) medications you gave incorrectly.
- Table C addresses the resources used for Stephanie Brown. Did you access the patient's chart, MAR, EPR, or Kardex as needed to make safe medication administration decisions?
- Did you check the patient's armband to verify her identity? Did you check whether your patient had any known allergies to medications? Were vital signs taken?

When you have finished reviewing the scorecard, click **Return to Evaluations** and then **Return to Menu**.

■ VITAL SIGNS

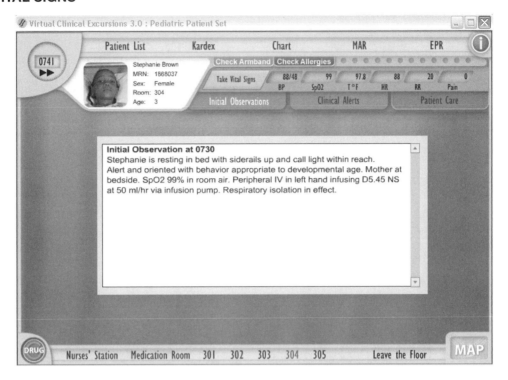

Vital signs, often considered the traditional "signs of life," include body temperature, heart rate, respiratory rate, blood pressure, oxygen saturation of the blood, and pain level.

Inside Stephanie Brown's room, click **Take Vital Signs**. (*Note:* If you are following this detailed tour step by step, you will need to **Restart the Program** from the Floor Menu, sign in again for Period of Care 1, and navigate to Room 304.) Collect vital signs for this patient and record them below. Note the time at which you collected each of these data. (*Remember:* You can take vital signs at any time. The data change over time to reflect the temporal changes you would find in a patient similar to Stephanie Brown.)

Vital Signs	Findings/Time
Blood pressure	
O$_2$ saturation	
Temperature	
Heart rate	
Respiratory rate	
Pain rating	

After you are done, click on the **EPR** icon located in the tool bar at the top of the screen. Your username and password are automatically provided. Click on **Login** to enter the EPR. To access Stephanie's records, click on the down arrow next to Patient and choose her room number, **304**. Select **Vital Signs** as the category. Next, in the empty time column on the far right, record the vital signs data you just collected in Stephanie's room. (*Note:* If you need help with this process, see page 16.) Now compare these findings with the data you collected earlier for this patient's vital signs. Use these earlier findings to establish a baseline for each of the vital signs.

    a.   Are any of the data you collected significantly different from the baseline for a particular vital sign?

        Circle One: Yes   No

    b.   If "Yes," which data are different?

■ PHYSICAL ASSESSMENT

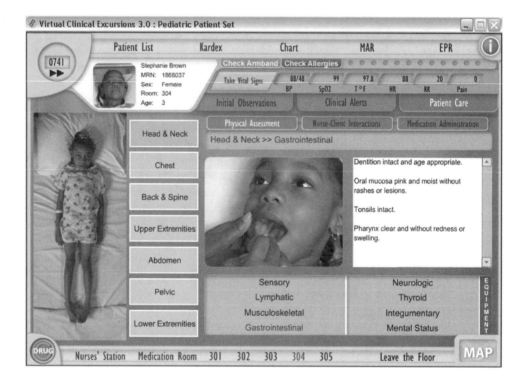

After you have finished examining the EPR for vital signs, click **Exit EPR** to return to Room 304. Click **Patient Care** and then **Physical Assessment**. Think about the information you received in the report at the beginning of this shift, as well as what you may have learned about this patient from the chart. Based on this, what area(s) of examination should you pay most attention to at this time? Is there any equipment you should be monitoring? Conduct a physical assessment of the body areas and systems that you consider priorities for Stephanie Brown. For example, select **Head & Neck**; then click on and assess **Sensory** and **Lymphatic**. Complete any other assessment(s) you think are necessary at this time. In the following table, record the data you collected during this examination.

Area of Examination	Findings
Head & Neck Sensory	
Head & Neck Lymphatic	

After you have finished collecting these data, return to the EPR. Compare the data that were already in the record with those you just collected.

   a. Are any of the data you collected significantly different from the baselines for this patient?

      Circle One: Yes   No

   b. If "Yes," which data are different?

■ NURSE-CLIENT INTERACTIONS

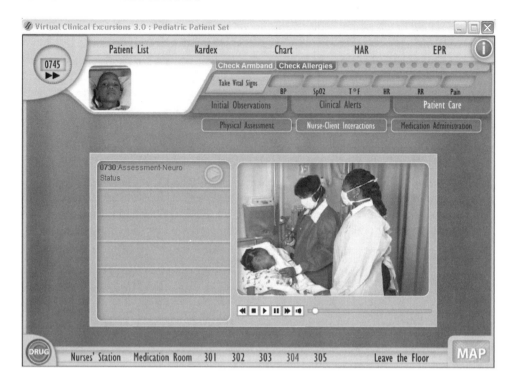

Click on **Patient Care** from inside Stephanie Brown's room (304). Now click on **Nurse-Client Interactions** to access a short video titled **Assessment—Neuro Status**, which is available for viewing at or after 0730 (based on the virtual clock in the upper left corner of your screen; see *Note* below). To begin the video, click on the white arrow next to its title. You will observe a nurse explaining her actions to Stephanie's mother. There are many variations of nursing practice, some exemplifying "best" practice and some not. Note whether the nurse in this interaction displays professional behavior and compassionate care. Are her words congruent with what is going on with the patient? Does this interaction "feel right" to you? If not, how would you handle this situation differently? Explain.

Note: If the video you wish to view is not listed, this means you have not yet reached the correct virtual time to view that video. Check the virtual clock; you may return to access the video once its designated time has occurred—as long as you do so within the same period of care. Or you can click on the fast-forward icon within the virtual clock to advance the time by 2-minute intervals. You will then need to click again on **Patient Care** and **Nurse-Client Interactions** to refresh the screen.

At least one Nurse-Client Interactions video is available during each period of care. Viewing these videos can help you learn more about what is occurring with a patient at a certain time and also prompt you to discern between nurse communications that are ideal and those that need improvement. Compassionate care and the ability to communicate clearly are essential components of delivering quality nursing care, and it is during your clinical time that you will begin to refine these skills.

COLLECTING AND EVALUATING DATA

Each of the activities you perform in the Patient Care environment generates a significant amount of assessment data. Remember that after you collect data, you can record your findings in the EPR. You can also review the EPR, patient's chart, videos, and MAR at any time. You will get plenty of practice collecting and then evaluating data in context of the patient's course.

Now, here's an important question for you:

> Did the previous sequence of exercises provide the most efficient way to assess Stephanie Brown?

For example, you went to the patient's room to get vital signs, then back to the EPR to enter data and compare your findings with extant data. Next, you went back to the patient's room to do a physical examination, then again back to the EPR to enter and review data. If this back-and-forth process of data collection and recording seemed inefficient, remember the following:

- Plan all of your nursing activities to maximize efficiency, while at the same time optimizing the quality of patient care. (Think about what data you might need before performing certain tasks. For example, do you need to check a heart rate before administering a cardiac medication or check an IV site before starting an infusion?)

- You collect a tremendous amount of data when you work with a patient. Very few people can accurately remember all these data for more than a few minutes. Develop efficient assessment skills, and record data as soon as possible after collecting them.

- Assessment data are only the starting point for the nursing process.

Make a clear distinction between these first exercises and how you actually provide nursing care. These initial exercises were designed to involve you actively in the use of different software components. This workbook focuses on sensible practices for implementing the nursing process in ways that ensure the highest-quality care of patients.

Most important, remember that a human being changes through time, and that these changes include both the physical and psychosocial facets of a person as a living organism. Think about this for a moment. Some patients may change physically in a very short time (a patient with emerging myocardial infarction) or more slowly (a patient with a chronic illness). Patients' overall physical and psychosocial conditions may improve or deteriorate. They may have effective coping skills and familial support, or they may feel alone and full of despair. In fact, each individual is a complex mix of physical and psychosocial elements, and at least some of these elements usually change through time.

Thus it is crucial that you *DO NOT* think of the nursing process as a simple one-time, five-step procedure consisting of assessment, nursing diagnosis, planning, implementation, and evaluation. Rather, the nursing process should be utilized as a creative and systematic approach to delivering nursing care. Furthermore, because all living organisms are constantly changing, we must apply the nursing process over and over. Each time we follow the nursing process for an individual patient, we refine our understanding of that patient's physical and psychosocial conditions based on collection and analysis of many different types of data. *Virtual Clinical Excursions—Pediatrics* will help you develop both the creativity and the systematic approach needed to become a nurse who is equipped to deliver the highest-quality care to all patients.

REDUCING MEDICATION ERRORS

Earlier in this detailed tour, you learned the basic steps of medication preparation and adminis-tration. The following simulations will allow you to practice those skills further—with an increased emphasis on reducing medication errors by using the Medication Scorecard to evalu-ate your work.

Sign in to work at Pacific View Regional Hospital for Period of Care 2. (*Note:* If you are already working with another patient or during another period of care, click on **Leave the Floor** and then **Restart the Program**; then sign in.)

From the Patient List, select Stephanie Brown. Then click on **Go to Nurses' Station**. Complete the following steps to prepare and administer medications to Stephanie Brown.

- Click on **Medication Room** on the tool bar at the bottom of your screen.
- Click on **MAR** and then on tab **304** to determine prn medications that have been ordered for Stephanie Brown. (*Note:* You may click on **Review MAR** at any time to verify the correct medication order. Always remember to check the patient name on the MAR to make sure you have the correct patient's record. You must click on the correct room number tab within the MAR.) Click on **Return to Medication Room** after reviewing the correct MAR.
- Click on **Unit Dosage** (or on the Unit Dosage cabinet); from the close-up view, click on drawer **304**.
- Select the medications you would like to administer. After each selection, click **Put Medica-tion on Tray**. When you are finished selecting medications, click **Close Drawer** and then **View Medication Room**.
- Click on **Automated System** (or on the Automated System unit itself). Click **Login**.
- On the next screen, specify the correct patient and drawer location.
- Select the medication you would like to administer and click on **Put Medication on Tray**. Repeat this process if you wish to administer other medications from the Automated System.
- When you are finished, click **Close Drawer** and **View Medication Room**.
- From the Medication Room, click on **Preparation** (or on the preparation tray).
- From the list of medications on your tray, highlight the correct medication to administer and click **Prepare**.
- This activates the Preparation Wizard. Supply any requested information; then click **Next**.
- Now select the correct patient to receive this medication and click **Finish**.
- Repeat the previous three steps until all medications that you want to administer are prepared.
- You can click on **Review Your Medications** and then on **Return to Medication Room** when ready. Once you are back in the Medication Room, go directly to Stephanie Brown's room by clicking on **304** at bottom of screen.
- Inside the patient's room, administer the medication, utilizing the six rights of medication administration. After you have collected the appropriate assessment data and are ready for administration, click **Patient Care** and then **Medication Administration**. Verify that the cor-rect patient and medication(s) appear in the left-hand window. Highlight the first medication you wish to administer; then click the down arrow next to Select. From the drop-down menu, select **Administer** and complete the Administration Wizard by providing any information requested. When the Wizard stops asking for information, click **Administer to Patient**. Specify **Yes** when asked whether this administration should be recorded in the MAR. Finally, click **Finish**.

■ SELF-EVALUATION

Now let's see how you did during your medication administration!

- Click on **Leave the Floor** at the bottom of your screen. From the Floor Menu, select **Look at Your Preceptor's Evaluation**. Then click on **Medication Scorecard**.

The following exercises will help you identify medication errors, investigate possible reasons for these errors, and reduce or prevent medication errors in the future.

1. Start by examining Table A. These are the medications you should have given to Stephanie Brown during this period of care. If each of the medications in Table A has a ✓ by it, then you made no errors. Congratulations!

If any medication has an X by it, then you made one or more medication errors.

Compare Tables A and B to determine which of the following types of errors you made: Wrong Dose, Wrong Route/Method/Site, or Wrong Time. Follow these steps:
   a. Find medications in Table A that were given incorrectly.
   b. Now see if those same medications are in Table B, which shows what you actually administered to Stephanie Brown.
   c. Comparing Tables A and B, match the Strength, Dose, Route/Method/Site, and Time for each medication you administered incorrectly.
   d. Then, using the form below, list the medications given incorrectly and mark the errors you made for each medication.

Medication	Strength	Dosage	Route	Method	Site	Time
	❑	❑	❑	❑	❑	❑
	❑	❑	❑	❑	❑	❑
	❑	❑	❑	❑	❑	❑
	❑	❑	❑	❑	❑	❑

2. To help you reduce future medication errors, consider the following list of possible reasons for errors.

- Did not check drug against MAR for correct medication, correct dose, correct patient, correct route, correct time, correct documentation.
- Did not check drug dose against MAR three times.
- Did not open the unit dose package in the patient's room.
- Did not correctly identify the patient using two identifiers.
- Did not administer the drug on time.
- Did not verify patient allergies.
- Did not check the patient's current condition or vital sign parameters.
- Did not consider why the patient would be receiving this drug.
- Did not question why the drug was in the patient's drawer.
- Did not check the physician's order and/or check with the pharmacist when there was a question about the drug or dose.
- Did not verify that no adverse effects had occurred from a previous dose.

Based on the list of possibilities you just reviewed, determine how you made each error and record the reason in the form below:

Medication	Reason for Error

3. Look again at Table B. Are there medications listed that are not in Table A? If so, you gave a medication to Stephanie Brown that she should not have received. Complete the following exercises to help you understand how such an error might have been made.

   a. Perhaps you gave a medication that was on Stephanie Brown's MAR for this period of care, without recognizing that a change had occurred in the patient's condition, which should have caused you to reconsider. Review patient records as necessary and complete the following form:

Medication	Possible Reasons Not to Give This Medication

   b. Another possibility is that you gave Stephanie Brown a medication that should have been given at a different time. Check her MAR and complete the form below to determine whether you made a Wrong Time error:

Medication	Given to Stephanie Brown at What Time	Should Have Been Given at What Time

c. Maybe you gave another patient's medication to Stephanie Brown. In this case, you made a Wrong Patient error. Check the MARs of other patients and use the form below to determine whether you made this type of error:

Medication	Given to Stephanie Brown	Should Have Been Given to

4. The Medication Scorecard provides some other interesting sources of information. For example, if there is a medication selected for Stephanie Brown but it was not given to her, there will be an X by that medication in Table A, but it will not appear in Table B. In that case, you might have given this medication to some other patient, which is another type of Wrong Patient error. To investigate further, look at Table D, which lists the medications you gave to other patients. See whether you can find any medications ordered for Stephanie Brown that were given to another patient by mistake. However, before you make any decisions, be sure to cross-check the MAR for other patients because the same medication may have been ordered for multiple patients. Use the following form to record your findings:

Medication	Should Have Been Given to Stephanie Brown	Given by Mistake to

5. Now take some time to review the medication exercises you just completed. Use the form below to create an overall analysis of what you have learned. Once again, record each of the medication errors you made, including the type of each error. Then, for each error you made, indicate specifically what you would do differently to prevent this type of error from occurring again.

Medication	Type of Error	Error Prevention Tactic

Submit this form to your instructor if required as a graded assignment, or simply use these exercises to improve your understanding of medication errors and how to reduce them.

Name: _____   Date: _____

The following icons are used throughout this workbook to help you quickly identify particular activities and assignments:

 Indicates a reading assignment—tells you which textbook chapter(s) you should read before starting each lesson

 Indicates a writing activity

 Marks the beginning of an interactive virtual hospital activity—signals you to open or return to your *Virtual Clinical Excursions—Pediatrics* simulation

 Indicates additional virtual hospital activity instructions

 Indicates questions and activities that require you to consult your textbook

 Indicates the approximate time required to complete an exercise

LESSON 1

Understanding Evidence-Based Practice

 Reading Assignment: Perspectives of Pediatric Nursing (Chapter 1)

Objectives:

1. Define the components of evidence-based practice (EBP).
2. Review appropriate search engines and websites to use as resources for pediatric nursing.
3. Define the levels of evidence used in EBP.

Exercise 1

Writing Activity

 30 minutes

1. The following table compares the steps of the nursing process with those of evidence-based practice. Fill in any missing steps or actions.

Nursing Process Steps	Actions	Evidence-Based Practice Steps	Actions
Assessment	Collects patient data		
Diagnosis			Collects information relevant to patient's identified problems and needs

Nursing Process Steps	Actions	Evidence-Based Practice Steps	Actions
		Analyzing evidence	Critically appraises published literature
Implementation	Initiates interventions identified in care plan		
	Evaluates patient's progress toward attainment of outcomes	Evaluating effectiveness	

2. List five examples of appropriate search engines and websites to use when researching each of the following topics:

Childhood obesity

End-of-life care for children

Head injury in children

3. List three organizations with websites that may include appropriate material for review of childhood immunizations.

4. What are PubMed and CINAHL? What are some differences and similarities between these two resources?

5. What is the AHRQ?

6. What types of information does the AHRQ provide? Why might this information be useful to the pediatric nurse?

7. Match each GRADE rating with its correct definition or recommendation.

GRADE Rating	**Definition**
_____ High	a. Evidence from RCTs with important limitations (inconsistent results, methodologic flaws, indirect evidence, or imprecise results) or unusually strong evidence from unbiased observational studies
_____ Moderate	
_____ Low	b. Evidence for at least one critical outcome from observational studies, from RCTs with serious flaws, or from indirect evidence
_____ Very low	
_____ Strong	c. Consistent evidence from well-performed randomized clinical trials (RCTs) or exceptionally strong evidence from unbiased observational studies
_____ Weak	
	d. Desirable effects closely balanced with undesirable effects
	e. Desirable effects clearly outweighing undesirable effects, or vice versa
	f. Evidence for at least one of the critical outcomes from unsystematic clinical observations or very indirect evidence

8. Provide two reasons why it is important to examine the quality of evidence when reviewing information on nursing care of children.

9. List the Institute of Medicine's six domains of Quality Patient Outcomes.

LESSON 2 _____

Understanding Head Injury

_____

👓 **Reading Assignment:** The Child with Cerebral Dysfunction (Chapter 37)

Patient: Tommy Douglas, Room 302

Objectives:

1. Evaluate the pathophysiology related to acute head trauma in children.
2. Perform a neurologic assessment on a child who has experienced a head injury.
3. Review medications given to a child who has experienced a head injury.

Exercise 1

✎ **Writing Activity**

 20 minutes

1. Describe the pathology of acute head injury in a child by matching the following terms and descriptions.

Term	Description
_____ Acceleration	a. Causes mass movement of the brain
_____ Deceleration	b. Causes bruising at the point of brain impact
_____ Subdural hematoma	c. Caused by unequal movement of the brain on impact
_____ Shearing forces	d. Bleeding between the dura and cerebrum
_____ Deformation	e. Causes greatest cerebral injury at the point of impact

2. What are the clinical symptoms of increased intracranial pressure (ICP) in a child Tommy Douglas' age?

3. What is the definition of cerebral perfusion pressure (CPP)? (*Hint:* The formula for CPP provides the definition and can be found in Chapter 37 of your textbook.)

4. Why is the concern for CPP important when caring for a patient with a head injury?

5. When cerebral blood flow is decreased, what symptoms frequently occur?

6. Which of the following vital sign changes are associated with brainstem injury following acute head trauma? Select all that apply.

_____ Rapid or intermittent respirations

_____ Wide fluctuations in pulse

_____ Widening pulse pressure

_____ Extreme fluctuations in blood pressure

_____ Elevated temperature

7. One of Tommy Douglas' nursing diagnoses is Risk for injury related to physical immobility, depressed sensorium, and intracranial pathology. List four nursing interventions for this nursing diagnosis specific to maintaining a stable ICP.

8. What is the expected outcome related to the nursing diagnosis presented in question 7?

Exercise 2

 Virtual Hospital Activity

 25 minutes

- Sign in to work at Pacific View Regional Hospital for Period of Care 1. (*Note:* If you are already in the virtual hospital from a previous exercise, click on **Leave the Floor** and then **Restart the Program** to get to the sign-in window.)
- From the Patient List, select Tommy Douglas (Room 302).
- Click on **Go to Nurses' Station**.
- Click on **Chart** and then on **302**.
- Click on **Emergency Department** and review the Admission Notes.
- While in the chart, also click on and review the **Nurse's Notes** and the **History and Physical.**

1. What caused Tommy Douglas' head injury?

2. Describe the sequence of events from the time of Tommy Douglas' injury to his arrival in the Emergency Department.

→ • Now click on **Expired MARs** and review Tommy Douglas' expired MAR for Sunday at 2300.

 • Next, click on **Physician's Orders** and review orders written in the Emergency Department.

 • For additional help with the following questions, consult the Drug Guide by first clicking on **Return to Nurses' Station** and then clicking on either the **Drug** icon in the lower left corner of the screen or the **Drug Guide** itself on the counter.

3. Based on your knowledge of head injury, why did Tommy Douglas receive mannitol?

4. Why did Tommy Douglas receive phenytoin?

5. Describe the sequence of events from Tommy Douglas' admission to the Emergency Department to his admission to your unit. (*Hint:* For help, check the Nurse's Notes, Physician's Notes, and Physician's Orders sections of the chart.)

6. List three interventions specific to the treatment of a child with a head injury that were performed before Tommy Douglas' arrival on your unit. (*Hint:* Access your Evolve student resources and view the nursing care plan for the unconscious child.)

LESSON 3

Assessing the Head-Injured Patient

Reading Assignment: Communication and Physical Assessment of the Child
(Chapter 6)
The Child with Cerebral Dysfunction (Chapter 37)

Patient: Tommy Douglas, Room 302

Objectives:

1. Perform a neurologic assessment on a child who has experienced a head injury.
2. Participate in the care of a comatose child.

Exercise 1

 Virtual Hospital Activity

 35 minutes

- Sign in to work at Pacific View Regional Hospital for Period of Care 1. (*Note:* If you are already in the virtual hospital from a previous exercise, click on **Leave the Floor** and then **Restart the Program** to get to the sign-in window.)
- From the Patient List, select Tommy Douglas (Room 302).
- Click on **Go to Nurses' Station**.
- Click on **Chart** and then on **302**.
- Click on **Emergency Department** and review the Admission Notes.
- Click on and review the **Nurse's Notes** and the **Physician's Notes**.

51

1. What are the major components of the Glasgow Coma Scale (GCS)?

 2. In the following table, provide a rationale for each test to explain its use in assessing the extent of Tommy Douglas' head injury. (*Hint:* You may want to review the Emergency Department Admission Notes, Nurse's Notes, Physician's Notes, and the EPR to determine the rationales. Also see Table 37-1 of your textbook.)

Diagnostic Test	Rationale for Test
Brain CT without contrast	
Skull x-ray	
Cervical spine x-ray (radiograph)	
Positron emission tomography (PET)	

Now let's assess Tommy Douglas' neurologic status over time since his admission to the Emergency Department. To do this, access and find neurologic assessment data in the following online resources, recording your findings in the table as instructed in question 3.

- In the patient's chart, click on **Emergency Department** and review the report for Sunday admission.
- Next, click on **Physician's Notes** and review the notes for Monday 0930 and Tuesday 1730.
- Click on **Return to Nurses' Station**.
- Select **EPR** and click on **Login**.
- Select **302** from the Patient drop-down menu and **Neurologic** from the Category drop-down menu.
- Review the neurologic findings for 0715 Wednesday.

3. In the table below, record the findings from your chart review of Tommy Douglas' neurologic status on Sunday, Monday, Tuesday, and Wednesday.

Neurologic Exam	Sunday Admission	Monday 0930	Tuesday 1730	Wednesday 0715
GCS: Total Score				
Pupils Right: Size				
Pupils Right: Reaction				
Pupils Left: Size				
Pupils Left: Reaction				
Cranial Nerves I-XII				
Orientation				
Perception and Cognition				
Mental Status				
Sensory				

- Click on **Exit EPR**.
- From the Nurses' Station, click on **Leave the Floor**.
- At the Floor Menu, select **Restart the Program**.
- Sign in for Period of Care 2.
- Again, select Tommy Douglas as your patient and click on **Go to Nurses' Station**.
- Now click on **EPR** and then on **Login**.
- Select **302** from the Patient drop-down menu and **Neurologic** from the Category drop-down menu.
- Review the results of the neurologic assessment recorded on Wednesday at 0800.

4. Complete the GCS form below, using the findings from Tommy Douglas' neurologic examination at 0800 Wednesday morning.

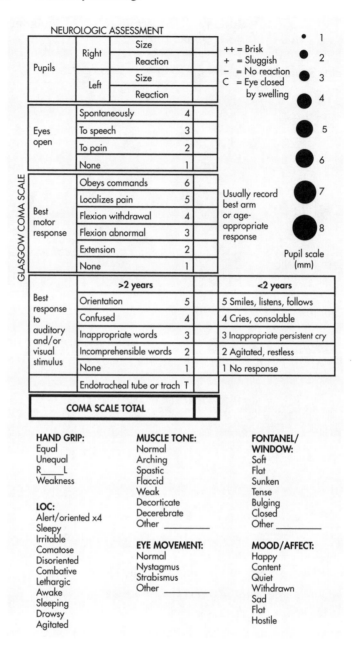

NEUROLOGIC ASSESSMENT

GLASGOW COMA SCALE

Pupils	Right	Size	
		Reaction	
	Left	Size	
		Reaction	

++ = Brisk
+ = Sluggish
− = No reaction
C = Eye closed by swelling

Eyes open	Spontaneously	4	
	To speech	3	
	To pain	2	
	None	1	

Best motor response	Obeys commands	6	
	Localizes pain	5	
	Flexion withdrawal	4	
	Flexion abnormal	3	
	Extension	2	
	None	1	

Usually record best arm or age-appropriate response

Pupil scale (mm)

Best response to auditory and/or visual stimulus	>2 years			<2 years
	Orientation	5		5 Smiles, listens, follows
	Confused	4		4 Cries, consolable
	Inappropriate words	3		3 Inappropriate persistent cry
	Incomprehensible words	2		2 Agitated, restless
	None	1		1 No response
	Endotracheal tube or trach	T		

COMA SCALE TOTAL | |

HAND GRIP:
Equal
Unequal
R____L
Weakness

LOC:
Alert/oriented x4
Sleepy
Irritable
Comatose
Disoriented
Combative
Lethargic
Awake
Sleeping
Drowsy
Agitated

MUSCLE TONE:
Normal
Arching
Spastic
Flaccid
Weak
Decorticate
Decerebrate
Other _____

EYE MOVEMENT:
Normal
Nystagmus
Strabismus
Other _____

FONTANEL/ WINDOW:
Soft
Flat
Sunken
Tense
Bulging
Closed
Other _____

MOOD/AFFECT:
Happy
Content
Quiet
Withdrawn
Sad
Flat
Hostile

5. How did Tommy Douglas' neurologic assessment results change from early in his admission to the Pediatric Intensive Care Unit (PICU) on Monday to his admission to the telemetry unit on Wednesday? Document your findings below. (*Hint:* Go to the chart and review the Nurse's Notes and Physician's Notes.)

Monday

Wednesday

6. Describe expected vital sign alterations in the head-injured child.

7. When caring for a critically ill patient such as Tommy Douglas, in what order would you conduct the following assessments? Number the assessments in order of priority from 1 to 4 (with 1 being the first assessment that you would conduct and 4 being the last).

_____ Check intravenous fluids and lines

_____ Perform a physical assessment

_____ Check ventilator settings

_____ Obtain vital sign results

Head Injury Management

 Reading Assignment: The Child with Endocrine Dysfunction (Chapter 38)

Patient: Tommy Douglas, Room 302

Objectives:

1. Analyze laboratory findings associated with acute head injury.
2. Review medications given to a child who has experienced a head injury.
3. Participate in the care of a comatose child.

Exercise 1

 Virtual Hospital Activity

🕐 25 minutes

- Sign in to work at Pacific View Regional Hospital for Period of Care 1. (*Note:* If you are already in the virtual hospital from a previous exercise, click on **Leave the Floor** and then **Restart the Program** to get to the sign-in window.)
- From the Patient List, select Tommy Douglas (Room 302).
- Click on **Go to Nurses' Station**.

1. Which of the symptoms below are commonly associated with diabetes insipidus? Select all that apply.

_____ Excessive urination

_____ Compensatory insatiable thirst

_____ Dehydration

_____ Electrolyte imbalance

_____ Circulatory collapse

To complete questions 2 through 6, use the following online resources as needed.

 • Click on **Chart** and then on **302**.
- Click on and review the **Nurse's Notes** and **Laboratory Reports**.
- Click on **Return to Nurses' Station**.
- Click on **EPR** and then on **Login**. Choose **302** from the Patient drop-down menu and review the results for the relevant available categories.
- Click on **Exit EPR**.
- Click on **MAR** and then on tab **302** for Tommy Douglas' records.

2. List three symptoms of diabetes insipidus that are manifested in Tommy Douglas. (*Note:* Indicate where/how you obtained your data, and be specific when you list symptoms—for example, "Vital signs: Tachycardia—HR greater than 120 bpm.")

3. What medication is being given to Tommy Douglas for the treatment of diabetes insipidus?

4. Describe this medication by completing the following table. (*Hint:* Use the Drug Guide as needed.)

Drug	Action	Availability	Dose and Frequency for Children

5. What medications are used as part of Tommy Douglas' treatment to assist with blood pressure management? (*Hint:* Check the MAR and the Physician's Orders.)

6. Describe these medications by completing the following table. (*Hint:* Use the Drug Guide as needed.)

Drug	Action	Availability	Dose and Frequency for Children

Acute Care Phase, Period of Care 1

 Reading Assignment: The Child with Cerebral Dysfunction (Chapter 37)

Patient: Tommy Douglas, Room 302

Objectives:

1. Perform a neurologic assessment on a child who has experienced a head injury.
2. Review medications given to a child who has experienced a head injury.
3. Participate in the care of a comatose child.
4. Interpret physical assessment findings related to a child whose condition is unstable.

Exercise 1

 Virtual Hospital Activity

35 minutes

- Sign in to work at Pacific View Regional Hospital for Period of Care 1. (*Note:* If you are already in the virtual hospital from a previous exercise, click on **Leave the Floor** and then **Restart the Program** to get to the sign-in window.)
- From the Patient List, select Tommy Douglas (Room 302).
- Click on **Go to Nurses' Station**.
- Click on **Chart** and then on **302**.
- Click on the **Physician's Orders** and review the orders written Wednesday morning.

1. List three orders written in Tommy Douglas' chart that are specific to the treatment of a child with a head injury.

• Click on **Return to Nurses' Station**.
   • Click on **EPR** and then on **Login**.
   • Select **302** from the Patient drop-down menu and **Vital Signs** from the Category drop-down menu. Review the given information.

 2. Evaluate Tommy Douglas' vital sign results on Wednesday at 0700 (just before this shift). Are they normal for his age or his condition at the time? (*Hint:* See the inside back cover of the textbook for vital sign values.)

Now take a current set of vital signs.

 • Click on **Exit EPR** and then on **302** at the bottom of the screen to go to Tommy Douglas' room.
   • Inside the room, click on **Take Vital Signs**.

3. Record Tommy Douglas' current vital signs below.

4. What changes are reflected in the current vital sign findings that indicate a need for prompt intervention?

5. What should be done immediately to prevent further neurologic and systemic deterioration in Tommy Douglas?

6. What should be given first to prevent systemic deterioration? Describe the initial intervention to correct the problem(s) identified in question 4.

➡ • Click on **Chart** and then on **302**.
   • Click on **Physician's Orders**.

7. Which of the orders written at 0730 Wednesday would have the most immediate effect on Tommy Douglas' blood pressure when implemented?

8. What additional physician order is written Wednesday morning at 0730 that is directly related to BP stabilization?

9. Before preparing and administering Tommy Douglas' medications, an appropriate weight must be obtained. What was his weight on admission? (*Hint:* See Nursing Admission in the chart.)

Answer the following questions in preparation for administering medication to Tommy Douglas.

10. Calculate the amount of norepinephrine that Tommy Douglas should receive based on his weight.

11. The infusion pump should be programmed to deliver _____ mL/hr to deliver the correct dose.

- Click on **Return to Room 302**.
- Click on **Medication Room** at the bottom of your screen.
- Click on **MAR** to determine which medications Tommy Douglas should receive at 0730. (*Note:* You may click on **Review MAR** at any time to verify the correct medication order. Remember to check the patient's name on the MAR to make sure you are viewing the correct record. You must click on the correct room number within the MAR.) Click on **Return to Medication Room** after reviewing the correct MAR.
- Click on **Unit Dosage** and then on drawer **302**.
- Click on the medication(s) you would like to administer. For each medication you select, click on **Put Medication on Tray**. When you are finished, click on **Close Drawer**.
- Click **View Medication Room**.
- Click on **Automated System** and then on **Login**.
- Select the correct patient and drawer according to the medication you want to administer. (*Hint:* The automated system is for controlled substances only.) Then click **Open Drawer**.
- Select the medication(s) you would like to administer, click **Put Medication on Tray**, and then **Close Drawer**.
- Click on **View Medication Room**.
- Begin the preparation process by clicking on **Preparation** at the top of the screen or clicking on the tray on the counter on the left side of the Medication Room.
- From the list of medications you put on the tray, select the medication you wish to administer and click **Prepare**.
- Supply any information requested by the Preparation Wizard and click **Next**.
- Choose the correct patient to administer this medication to and click **Finish**.
- Repeat the above three steps until all medications that you want to administer are prepared.
- You can click on **Review Your Medications** and then **Return to Medication Room** when ready.

Before you administer Tommy Douglas' medications, you must first check his existing intravenous lines and the fluids being administered through these lines.

- Click on **EPR** and then on **Login**.
- Select **302** from the Patient drop-down menu and **IV** from the Category drop-down menu.
- Review the data recorded on Wednesday at 0700.
- Now click on **Exit EPR** and then on **Chart**.
- Click on **302**.
- Select the **Physician's Orders** tab.
- Find the orders for Wednesday at 0600 and review to learn more about the fluids being infused through Tommy Douglas' IV lines.

12. Complete the following table to review the types of lines Tommy Douglas has and the fluids infusing through each line at 0700 on Wednesday.

Type of Intravenous Line	Location of Intravenous Line	Type of Fluid Infusing and Rationale for Using This Intravenous Line
Central venous line		
Peripheral line		
Arterial line		

 • Now go to Tommy Douglas' room to administer his medication(s).
- Click on **Return to Medication Room** and then on **302** at the bottom of the screen.
- Inside the room, click on **Patient Care** and then on **Medication Administration**.
- Next to the medication(s) you want to give, click on **Select** and choose **Administer** from the drop-down menu.
- Complete the Administration Wizard questions; then click on **Administer to Patient**.
- Specify **Yes** to document this to the MAR.
- Finally, click **Finish**.
- Still in his room, click on **Take Vital Signs**.

13. What are Tommy Douglas' current vital signs?

14. What vital signs would you assess to evaluate the effectiveness of the medication administered in question 6?

• Click on **Patient Care** and then on **Nurse-Client Interactions**.
 • Select and view the video titled **0800: Intervention—Stabilizing BP**. (*Note:* Check the virtual clock to see whether enough time has elapsed. You can use the fast-forward feature to advance the time by 2-minute intervals if the video is not yet available. Then click again on **Patient Care** and **Nurse-Client Interactions** to refresh the screen.)

In this video, the nurse informs Tommy Douglas' parents that she will be giving him fluids to help stabilize his blood pressure. Let's jump forward in virtual time to evaluate the effectiveness of this intervention.

 • Click on **Leave the Floor**.
 • From the Floor Menu, select **Restart the Program**.
 • Sign in for Period of Care 2.
 • Choose Tommy Douglas as your patient; then click on **Go to Nurses' Station**.
 • From the Nurses' Station, click on **EPR** and then on **Login**.
 • Select **302** from the Patient drop-down menu and **Vital Signs** from the Category drop-down menu.
 • Use the left-pointing blue arrow at the bottom of the screen to move back to the data recorded on Wednesday at 0900.

15. What was Tommy Douglas' BP at 0900 after the normal saline bolus was administered? Did his blood pressure improve as a result of this intervention?

Acute Care Phase, Period of Care 2

 Reading Assignment: The Child with Cerebral Dysfunction (Chapter 37)

Patient: Tommy Douglas, Room 302

Objectives:

1. Interpret physical assessment findings related to a child whose condition is unstable.
2. Analyze laboratory findings associated with acute head injury.
3. Observe interactions between health care providers and parents experiencing the loss of a child.

Exercise 1

 Virtual Hospital Activity

🕐 20 minutes

- Sign in to work at Pacific View Regional Hospital for Period of Care 2. (*Note:* If you are already in the virtual hospital from a previous exercise, click on **Leave the Floor** and then **Restart the Program** to get to the sign-in window.)
- From the Patient List, select Tommy Douglas (Room 302).
- Click on **Get Report.**
- Click on **Go to Nurses' Station**.
- Click on **302** at the bottom of the screen.
- Inside Tommy Douglas' room, click on **Take Vital Signs**.

1. Document Tommy Douglas' current vital signs in the table below. Also, document these findings in the EPR. (*Hint:* If you need to review the steps for entering data in the EPR, see pp. 13-14 in the **Getting Started** section of this workbook.)

Vital Sign	Findings
Temperature (F)	
Systolic pressure	
Diastolic pressure	
BP mode of measurement	
Heart rate	
Respiratory rate	
SpO_2 (%)	

→ • While you are still in Tommy Douglas' room, review the **Initial Observations**.
   • Next, click on **Patient Care** and then on **Physical Assessment**.
   • Choose the various physical assessment areas (yellow buttons) and appropriate subcategories (green buttons) as needed to complete the table in question 2.

2. Below and on the next page, record your findings from the physical assessment.

Assessment Area	Findings
General Appearance	
HEENT	
Pulmonary	
Cardiovascular	

Assessment Area	Findings
Gastrointestinal	
Genitourinary	
Musculoskeletal	
Neurologic	

→ • Now click on **Chart** and then on **302**.
  • Click on **Physician's Orders** and review the orders for Wednesday 1100.
  • Click on **Laboratory Reports** and review the findings for Wednesday morning.

3. In the table below record Tommy Douglas' CBC findings for Wednesday morning. Place an asterisk (*) after any abnormal findings.

Hematology Laboratory Test	Findings
Hemoglobin	
Hematocrit	
Platelets	

4. What has the physician ordered for Tommy Douglas at 1100?

5. What is the most likely rationale for this order, given Tommy Douglas' laboratory values at 1100?

6. What other medications are being infused at this same time?

➡ • Still in the Laboratory Reports section of the chart, review Tommy Douglas' arterial blood gas values for 0700 on Wednesday.

7. Record Tommy Douglas' ABG results in the following table.

Arterial Blood Gas Test	Findings—Wednesday 0700
PaO_2	
$PaCO_2$	
pH	
Bicarbonate	

8. Select the type of acid-base imbalance represented by Tommy Douglas' 0700 ABG results.

    _____ Metabolic alkalosis

    _____ Respiratory alkalosis

    _____ Respiratory acidosis

    _____ Metabolic acidosis

9. Which of the following statements is true regarding acid-base imbalance?
    a. Respiratory acidosis is reflected by increased plasma pH and decreased plasma $PaCO_2$.
    b. Metabolic alkalosis is reflected by decreased plasma pH and decreased plasma $PaCO_2$.
    c. Metabolic acidosis is reflected by decreased plasma pH and increased plasma $PaCO_2$.
    d. Respiratory alkalosis is reflected by increased plasma pH and decreased plasma $PaCO_2$.

→ • Review the **Physician's Orders** written for Tommy Douglas at 0820 on Wednesday.

10. What medication was ordered for Tommy Douglas at this time?

11. What is the most likely rationale for administering this medication to Tommy Douglas?

12. What is the normal dose range for this medication when administered to a child Tommy Douglas' age?

13. Based on his weight, did Tommy Douglas receive a therapeutic dose of this medication?

14. Below, record Tommy Douglas' ABG results for Wednesday at 0900. (*Hint:* Find these in the Laboratory Reports in the chart.)

Arterial Blood Gas Test	Findings—Wednesday 0900
PaO_2	
$PaCO_2$	
pH	
Bicarbonate	

15. What evidence is there (if any) that the medication identified in question 10 was effective?

- Click on **Return to Room 302**.
- Click on **Patient Care** and then on **Nurse-Client Interactions**.
- Select and view the video titled **1115: The Family (Care) Conference**. (*Note:* Check the virtual clock to see whether enough time has elapsed. You can use the fast-forward feature to advance the time by 2-minute intervals if the video is not yet available. Then click again on **Patient Care** and **Nurse-Client Interactions** to refresh the screen.)
- After viewing the video, click on **Chart** and then on **302**.
- Review the **Physician's Notes** and **Consultations**.

16. What specific tests did the physicians review with Tommy Douglas' parents?

17. What specific findings on physical examination were listed in the consultation notes that concurred with the diagnosis of brain death?

18. What is the caloric test? (*Hint:* See Chapter 37 in your textbook.)

 • Click on **Return to Room 302**.
• Click on **Patient Care** and then on **Nurse-Client Interactions**.
• Select and view the video titled **1130: Decision—Organ Donation**. (*Note:* Check the virtual clock to see whether enough time has elapsed. You can use the fast-forward feature to advance the time by 2-minute intervals if the video is not yet available. Then click again on **Patient Care** and **Nurse-Client Interactions** to refresh the screen.)

19. What was discussed with Tommy Douglas' parents in the 1130 conference?

20. Who was present at the 1115 and 1130 family care conferences?

21. Why is a multidisciplinary team approach important for Tommy Douglas' family?

Acute Care Phase, Period of Care 3

 Reading Assignment: Family-Centered End-of-Life Care (Chapter 23)
The Child with Cerebral Dysfunction (Chapter 37)

Patient: Tommy Douglas, Room 302

Objectives:

1. Interpret physical assessment findings related to a child whose condition is unstable.
2. Analyze laboratory findings associated with acute head injury.
3. Describe the diagnostic evaluation necessary to confirm brain death in a child.
4. Observe interactions between health care providers and parents experiencing the loss of a child.

Exercise 1

 Virtual Hospital Activity

30 minutes

- Sign in to work at Pacific View Regional Hospital for Period of Care 3. (*Note:* If you are already in the virtual hospital from a previous exercise, click on **Leave the Floor** and then **Restart the Program** to get to the sign-in window.)
- From the Patient List, select Tommy Douglas (Room 302).
- Click on **Go to Nurses' Station**.
- Click on **302** at the bottom of the screen to go to Tommy Douglas' room.
- Click on **Take Vital Signs**.
- Document Tommy Douglas' 1500 vital signs results in the **EPR**. (*Hint:* If you need help entering data in the EPR, see pp. 13-14 in the **Getting Started** section of this workbook.)
- When you have finished entering these data, click on **Exit EPR**.
- Now click on **Chart** and then on **302**.
- Click on **Physician's Orders**.

1. Why were new orders written at this time?

 • Review Tommy Douglas' chart as needed to answer question 2.

2. In the left column below, list the tests used to establish brain death. In the right column, summarize the results of these tests for Tommy Douglas.

Diagnostic Test	Findings for Tommy Douglas

 • Click on **Return to Room 302**.
• Click on **Patient Care** and then on **Physical Assessment**.
• Click on **Head & Neck**.
• Click on **Neurologic** and complete a neurologic assessment on Tommy Douglas.
• Now click on **EPR** and then on **Login**.
• Select **302** from the Patient drop-down menu and **Neurologic** from the Category drop-down menu.
• Review the findings for Wednesday at 1400.

3. Based on your review of the EPR and the in-room neurologic assessment, record Tommy Douglas' neurologic findings for Wednesday 1400-1430 in the table below and on the next page.

Neurologic Exam	Exam Findings 1400-1430
Glasgow Coma Scale: Eyes	
Glasgow Coma Scale: Verbal	
Glasgow Coma Scale: Motor	
Glasgow Coma Scale: Total Score	
Pupils Right: Size	
Pupils Right: Reaction	
Pupils Left: Size	
Pupils Left: Reaction	

Neurologic Exam	Exam Findings 1400-1430

Cranial Nerves I-XII

Orientation

Speech

Cognitive and Perceptual

Mental Status

Sensation

- Click on **Exit EPR**.
- Click on **Chart** and then on **302**.
- Click on and review the **Physician's Notes** and **Consultations.**

4. Are your physical examination findings consistent with what you reviewed in the Physician's Notes and Consultations?

5. What is important for the nurse to know when caring for a patient whose organs will soon be donated? (*Hint:* See Chapter 23 of your textbook.)

- Click on **Return to Room 302**.
- Once again, observe Tommy Douglas' vital signs by clicking on **Take Vital Signs**.

6. Record Tommy Douglas' current vital signs below.

Assessment	Findings

Temperature (F)

Systolic pressure

Diastolic pressure

BP mode of measurement

Heart rate

Respiratory

SpO$_2$ (%)

7. Tommy Douglas' current vital signs indicate what continuing problem(s)?

 • Click on **Patient Care** and then on **Nurse-Client Interactions**.
 • Select and view the video titled **1500: Nurse-Family Communication**. (*Note:* Check the virtual clock to see whether enough time has elapsed. You can use the fast-forward feature to advance the time by 2-minute intervals if the video is not yet available. Then click again on **Patient Care** and **Nurse-Client Interactions** to refresh the screen.)

8. What was reinforced by the nurse during this conversation?

9. Why was it important for the nurse in the video interaction to discuss ways for the family to remember Tommy Douglas?

• Now click on and view the video titled **1515: The Grieving Family** to observe the specialist/family interaction. (*Note:* Check the virtual clock to see whether enough time has elapsed. You can use the fast-forward feature to advance the time by 2-minute intervals if the video is not yet available. Then click again on **Patient Care** and **Nurse-Client Interactions** to refresh the screen.)

10. Describe the role of a child-life specialist and why this individual is an appropriate choice to meet with Tommy Douglas' siblings.

Providing Support for Families Experiencing the Loss of a Child

Reading Assignment: Family-Centered End-of-Life Care (Chapter 23)

Patient: Tommy Douglas, Room 302

Objectives:

1. Provide nursing care for the child and family at the end of life.
2. Participate in the multidisciplinary care of the child and family at the end of life.

Exercise 1

Virtual Hospital Activity

45 minutes

- Sign in to work at Pacific View Regional Hospital for Period of Care 2. (*Note:* If you are already in the virtual hospital from a previous exercise, click on **Leave the Floor** and then **Restart the Program** to get to the sign-in window.)
- From the Patient List, select Tommy Douglas (Room 302).
- Click on **Get Report** and read the report.
- Click on **Go to Nurses' Station**.
- Click on **302** at the bottom of the screen to go to Tommy Douglas' room.

1. Complete the following table regarding important principles for communicating with families and effective techniques that should be used.

Communication Approach	Effective Communication Techniques

• Click on **Patient Care** and then on **Nurse-Client Interactions**.

• Select and view the video titled **1115: The Family (Care) Conference**. (*Note:* Check the virtual clock to see whether enough time has elapsed. You can use the fast-forward feature to advance the time by 2-minute intervals if the video is not yet available. Then click again on **Patient Care** and **Nurse-Client Interactions** to refresh the screen.)

2. Complete the table below by identifying what you observed in the family care conference, including those communication techniques that were missing or not fully executed.

Communication Approach	Communication Techniques

3. What are the ages of Tommy Douglas' siblings?

4. Based on the ages of Tommy Douglas' siblings, describe below preschool and school-age children's typical reactions to death and identify possible interventions for support of Tommy Douglas' siblings.

Preschool children

School-age children

• Click on **Chart** and then on **302**.

• Click on **Consultations** and read the Social Services Consult, Pastoral Consult, and the Child-Life Consult.

5. List at least four interventions found in the consultants' plans that provide an understanding of the health care roles of the following: chaplain, social worker, and child-life specialist. Identify the interventions performed by each specific health care professional in this scenario.

 6. Identify at least three strategies discussed in the textbook that can assist nurses and other health care professionals to cope with the loss of a child in their care. (*Hint:* See the section on Coping with Stress in Chapter 23 in your textbook.)

7. What is nursing burnout? What strategies might you use to prevent this from happening to you?

Developing an EBP Summary Review: Pain Management for Children Who Are Dying

∽ Reading Assignment: Family-Centered End-of-Life Care (Chapter 23)
The Child with Cerebral Dysfunction (Chapter 37)

Patient: Tommy Douglas, Room 302

Objectives:

1. Describe the critical elements of an EBP review summary.
2. Develop an EBP summary review of pain management for children who are dying.

Before beginning this lesson, complete Lessons 2 through 8. These lessons focus on Tommy Douglas, a child who was admitted to the hospital because of traumatic head injury that has left him comatose. Tommy Douglas will not recover from the head injury and will die soon. Lessons 2 through 8 provided an overview of the care required for a patient with severe head injury. This lesson will give you an opportunity to explore the research on pain experiences of dying children. Although Tommy Douglas' situation does not allow us to evaluate the presence of pain in a dying child, this review will provide you with an understanding of the pain experiences of dying children.

Exercise 1

Writing Activity

60 minutes

Before you begin developing your EBP summary review, remember the following guidelines:

- Begin by establishing the purpose of the review.
- Next, think about the key terms or words you will use to search the literature.
- Once you decide on your search terms, think about where you will search.
- What organizations might have websites that provide information on this subject?
- What national agencies might have studies that review the information? (Remember to search on the Cochrane Collaboration and AHRQ websites.)
- Remember to search both nursing and medical literature.

- Once your search is completed, critically review each article and evaluate the evidence. In a sentence or two, summarize the study. Include the study purpose, sample, design, procedures, and findings.
- Apply the findings to nursing practice. What recommendations can you make to clinical practice?
- In the final box of the EBP summary review, include all the references you used in the summary. Be sure you write these in an appropriate reference style for your nursing program.

1. Using the guidelines just summarized, complete the following EBP summary review of the pain experience of children who are dying.

Ask the Question

Question

Search the Evidence

Databases Searched

Search Strategies

Critically Analyze the Evidence

Provide a concise synopsis of each article relevant to the subject.

Summary of Findings

Apply Evidence Recommendations

What nursing implications can be recommended based on your summary of the findings?

References **List at least four references you used in your review.**

LESSON 10
Anorexia Nervosa: History and Physical Examination

 Reading Assignment: Behavioral Health Problems of Adolescence (Chapter 21)

Patient: Tiffany Sheldon, Room 305

Objectives:

1. Participate in the care of the adolescent with anorexia nervosa.
2. Identify the early signs of anorexia nervosa.

Exercise 1

 Virtual Hospital Activity

25 minutes

- Sign in to work at Pacific View Regional Hospital for Period of Care 1. (*Note:* If you are already in the virtual hospital from a previous exercise, click on **Leave the Floor** and then **Restart the Program** to get to the sign-in window.)
- From the Patient List, select Tiffany Sheldon (Room 305).
- Click on **Go to Nurses' Station**.
- Click on **Chart** and then on **305**.
- Click on **Emergency Department** and review the record.

1. Describe Tiffany Sheldon's past illness history leading up to her Emergency Department visit.

2. List the three treatment goals for patients with anorexia nervosa. (*Hint:* Review Chapter 21 in your textbook.)

→ • While still in the chart, click on **Nursing Admission**.

3. Review the Nursing Admission and list three family stressors found in Tiffany Sheldon's family.

→ • Now click on **Physician's Orders**.
• Note Tiffany Sheldon's medical diagnosis documented on the Physician's Orders for 0600 Wednesday.
• Click on **Return to Nurses' Station**.
• Click on **305** at the bottom of your screen to enter Tiffany Sheldon's room.
• Click on **Patient Care**.
• Click on **Physical Assessment**.
• Perform a focused physical assessment on Tiffany Sheldon by clicking on the various body systems in the yellow boxes.

4. List six findings from the physical assessment that relate to Tiffany Sheldon's diagnosis of malnutrition.

→ • Click on **Chart** and then on **305** to access Tiffany Sheldon's chart once again.

5. Based on the Emergency Department admission data and Tiffany Sheldon's past and present health history, list three appropriate nursing diagnoses with the etiology statement included.

6. What was Tiffany Sheldon's weight on admission to the Emergency Department?

7. What is Tiffany Sheldon's height? (*Hint:* Review the Nursing Admission in the chart.)

8. Review the CDC growth chart on the next page. Based on this chart, Tiffany Sheldon is in what percentile for weight? (*Hint:* Body mass index [BMI] information can be found in Chapter 21 and in Appendix B of your textbook.)

9. What is Tiffany Sheldon's ideal body weight? (*Hint:* 50th percentile for age.)

10. Tiffany Sheldon's current body weight is what percentage of her ideal body weight?

11. What was Tiffany Sheldon's BMI prior to her diagnosis with anorexia nervosa (at 12 years of age)? What was her BMI on admission? Identify the percentile of each of her BMI scores.

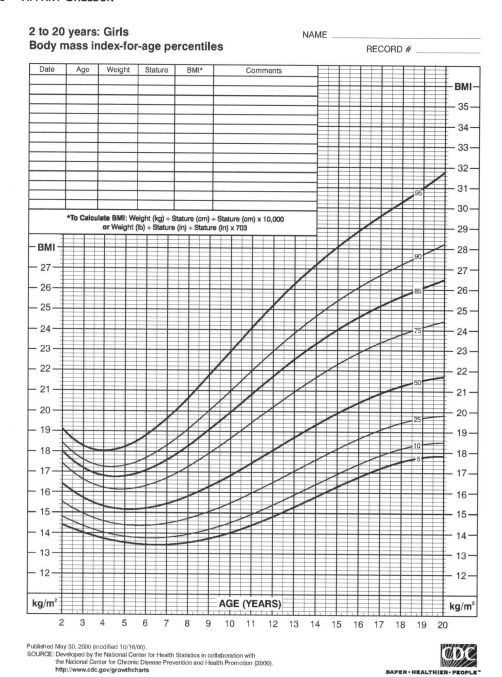

2 to 20 years: Girls
Body mass index-for-age percentiles

NAME _____

RECORD # _____

Published May 30, 2000 (modified 10/16/00).
SOURCE: Developed by the National Center for Health Statistics in collaboration with
the National Center for Chronic Disease Prevention and Health Promotion (2000).
http://www.cdc.gov/growthcharts

 12. Based on Tiffany Sheldon's present health history and current assessment findings, list two criteria from Box 21-8 in your textbook that confirm the need for her present hospitalization.

Pathophysiology of Anorexia Nervosa

 Reading Assignment: Behavioral Health Problems of Adolescence (Chapter 21)

Patient: Tiffany Sheldon, Room 305

Objectives:

1. Participate in the care of the adolescent with anorexia nervosa.
2. Identify the early signs of anorexia nervosa.
3. Describe the DSM-IV diagnostic criteria for anorexia nervosa in relation to the case study patient.
4. Distinguish between the two different types of anorexia nervosa.
5. Describe physical and behavioral characteristics of the adolescent with anorexia nervosa.

Exercise 1

 Virtual Hospital Activity

15 minutes

- Sign in to work at Pacific View Regional Hospital for Period of Care 1. (*Note:* If you are already in the virtual hospital from a previous exercise, click on **Leave the Floor** and then **Restart the Program** to get to the sign-in window.)
- From the Patient List, select Tiffany Sheldon (Room 305).
- Click on **Go to Nurses' Station**.
- Click on **Chart** and then on **305**.
- Click on **History and Physical** and review the record.

 1. What are the early signs of anorexia nervosa that Tiffany Sheldon reportedly exhibits? (*Hint:* See Box 21-9 in your textbook.)

2. Based on the History and Physical, which type of anorexia nervosa does Tiffany Sheldon have? Explain your answer based on her recent history as reported by her mother. (*Hint:* See Box 21-6 in your textbook.)

3. The incidence of anorexia nervosa is highest in which of the following age groups?
   a. 11-13 years
   b. 14-16 years
   c. 14-19 years
   d. 20-23 years

4. What are some personality characteristics commonly found in children with anorexia nervosa?
   a. Perfectionists, academically high achievers, conforming, and conscientious
   b. Fearful, dependent, and controlling
   c. Goal-oriented, physically active, with erratic behaviors
   d. All of the above

5. All of the following are psychologic characteristics of anorexia nervosa *except*:
   a. Pursuit of thinness
   b. Fear of fatness
   c. Disordered body perception
   d. Response to traumatic or personal life events
   e. Response to teasing, life changes
   f. Sequelae of infectious diseases

For questions 6 through 12, indicate whether each statement is true or false. If a statement is false, provide a rationale.

6. _____ Young people involved in competitive sports or activities such as ballet and gymnastics are also at risk for unsafe weight control practices and eating disorders such as anorexia nervosa. (True/False)

7. _____ Anorexia nervosa is more common in females. (True/False)

8. _____ Females typically have a more difficult clinical course than males who are diagnosed with anorexia nervosa. (True/False)

9. _____ Physical changes associated with anorexia nervosa are reversible with adequate nutrition and leave no sequelae. (True/False)

10. _____ It is rare for patients with anorexia nervosa to die from associated complications. (True/False)

11. _____ Poor outcomes in the individual with anorexia nervosa are associated with existing disturbed family relationships, a strong compulsion to exercise, and a prolonged course of illness. (True/False)

12. _____ Patients with an eating disorder such as anorexia nervosa rarely have associated psychiatric problems. (True/False)

12

Anorexia Nervosa: Clinical Signs and Symptoms

∞ **Reading Assignment:** Communication and Physical Assessment of the Child
(Chapter 6)
Balance and Imbalance of Body Fluids (Chapter 28)

Patient: Tiffany Sheldon, Room 305

Objectives:

1. Identify the physical assessment characteristics of a child with anorexia nervosa.
2. Recognize potentially life-threatening physical assessment findings in the child with anorexia nervosa.
3. Identify diagnostic laboratory values indicative of dehydration.

Exercise 1

Virtual Hospital Activity

30 minutes

- Sign in to work at Pacific View Regional Hospital for Period of Care 1. (*Note:* If you are already in the virtual hospital from a previous exercise, click on **Leave the Floor** and then **Restart the Program** to get to the sign-in window.)
- From the Patient List, select Tiffany Sheldon (Room 305).
- Click on **Go to Nurses' Station**.
- Click on **Chart** and then on **305**.
- Click on **Emergency Department** and review the record.

1. The Review of Systems in the Emergency Department revealed the findings in the right column below. Match each finding with the corresponding body system.

Body System		Finding
_____	Integumentary	a. Upper and lower extremity weakness
_____	Cardiovascular	b. 4-second capillary refill and 1+ pedal edema
_____	Genitourinary	c. Decreased skin turgor and dry skin
_____	Gastrointestinal	d. Constipation
_____	Neuromuscular	e. Decreased urine output

2. List the clinical findings of the physical examination documented by the nurse and physician in the Emergency Department.

3. Identify initial clinical findings in the Emergency Department Record that require immediate attention.

4. Describe the most likely cause of the findings you identified in the previous question, as well as the significance of the findings. (*Hint:* See the section on Dehydration in Chapter 28 of your textbook.)

- Click on **Return to Nurses' Station**.
- Click on **305** at the bottom of your screen to go to Tiffany Sheldon's room.
- Click on **Patient Care** and then on **Nurse-Client Interactions**.
- Select and view the video titled **0730: Initial Assessment**. (*Note:* Check the virtual clock to see whether enough time has elapsed. You can use the fast-forward feature to advance the time by 2-minute intervals if the video is not yet available. Then click again on **Patient Care** and **Nurse-Client Interactions** to refresh the screen.)

5. In the video, what assessment does the nurse perform related to Tiffany Sheldon's cardio-vascular status? What is the clinical significance of making this assessment and the manner in which the nurse performs it?

6. What else does the nurse ask Tiffany Sheldon in the video interaction that represents cardio-vascular assessment?

• Click on **Chart** and then on **305**.
• Select **Laboratory Reports**.
• Review the findings documented in the Emergency Department on Wednesday at 0530.

7. Below, record Tiffany Sheldon's laboratory results obtained in the Emergency Department. For each test, also provide the normal range of values for a child her age (14). (*Hint:* See Appendix C in your textbook.)

Test	Tiffany Sheldon's Result	Normal Range
Glucose		
Sodium		
Potassium		
Chloride		
Creatinine—serum		
BUN		
Calcium—serum, total		
Protein—serum		
Albumin		

8. Identify a laboratory value from Tiffany Sheldon's complete blood count that is significant in the diagnosis of dehydration.

9. Tiffany Sheldon's physician has ordered specific gravity every void. What does specific gravity measure? What is the significance of this clinical finding in relation to the patient's clinical status?

→ • Now click on and review the initial **Physician's Orders**.

10. Tiffany Sheldon is being treated for dehydration. What other laboratory tests have been ordered to assess and monitor the status of her dehydration?
    a. Albumin, protein, and alkaline phosphatase
    b. HCG urinalysis and specific gravity
    c. Glucose, phosphorus, calcium, and magnesium
    d. BUN, creatinine, Chem 7 (basic metabolic panel)

11. What is the purpose of obtaining a urine HCG on Tiffany Sheldon? What does the test reveal?

12. Tiffany Sheldon has been diagnosed with malnutrition. Which of the following laboratory tests are ordered to assess and monitor her malnutrition?
    a. Serum VDRL, specific gravity, and alkaline phosphatase
    b. Protein, albumin, glucose, and alkaline phosphatase
    c. Protein, calcium, ALT, and AST
    d. Chem 7 (basic metabolic panel), protein, and BUN

13. Tiffany Sheldon has been diagnosed with bradycardia. Which of the following laboratory tests assess and monitor her cardiac function?
    a. BUN, creatinine, protein, and glucose
    b. Chem 7 (basic metabolic panel), VDRL, specific gravity, and alkaline phosphatase
    c. Chem 7 (basic metabolic panel), phosphorus, calcium, and magnesium
    d. ALT, AST, urine specific gravity, and protein

→ • Next, click on **Nursing Admission** and review.

14. Upon admission, what risks were assessed for Tiffany Sheldon? Select all that apply.

    _____ Risk for infection

    _____ Risk for hypertension

    _____ Risk for falls

    _____ Risk for impaired tissue integrity

15. What are the underlying causes of these assessed risks?
    a. Poor nutrition, electrolyte imbalance, and muscle wasting
    b. Poor nutrition, depression, and too much exercise
    c. Amenorrhea, electrolyte imbalance, and depression
    d. Muscle wasting, depression, and too much exercise

16. What is the best explanation for the finding of lanugo in Tiffany Sheldon's physical exam?
    a. Hair follicles are starved of the appropriate nutrition needed to produce healthy hair.
    b. It is the result of cold intolerance in attempt to warm the body.
    c. It is secondary to cardiac insufficiency.
    d. All of the above explain Tiffany Sheldon's finding of lanugo.

17. Rapid weight gain, also referred to as refeeding syndrome, should be avoided in patients with anorexia nervosa because of which of the following? Select all that apply.

    _____ It has been associated with severe metabolic abnormalities.

    _____ Cardiovascular overload has led to death in patients with anorexia nervosa.

    _____ Patients with anorexia nervosa are fearful of gaining weight.

    _____ Patients with anorexia nervosa have a distorted body image.

18. Urinary tract problems are frequent in patients with anorexia nervosa, including the presence of ketones and proteins in the urine. What is the most likely cause of these findings?
    a. Low body temperature
    b. Fat and protein breakdown
    c. Decreased cardiac output

19. Tiffany Sheldon complains of problems with constipation. This finding is related to which of the following? Select all that apply.

    _____ Delayed gastric emptying

    _____ Decreased fluid intake

    _____ Muscle wasting

    _____ Reduced intestinal motility

20. Tiffany Sheldon does *not* have which of the following physical symptoms of anorexia nervosa? Select all that apply.

_____ Lowered body temperature

_____ Bradycardia

_____ Decreased blood pressure

_____ Cold intolerance

_____ Headaches

_____ Vomiting

_____ Secondary amenorrhea

21. What best explains the finding of edema on admission?

22. List two laboratory tests from question 7 for which the values are helpful in evaluating the malnourished patient.

Management of Anorexia Nervosa

—————————————————————————————————————

Reading Assignment: Behavioral Health Problems of Adolescence (Chapter 21)
The Child with Cardiovascular Dysfunction (Chapter 34)

Patient: Tiffany Sheldon, Room 305

Objectives:

1. Participate in the care of the adolescent with anorexia nervosa.
2. Discuss the special care needs of the adolescent with anorexia nervosa.
3. Identify the contents and goal of the behavioral or "eating" contract.
4. Describe the role of the multidisciplinary health care team in the management of anorexia nervosa.

Exercise 1

 Writing Activity

 5 minutes

1. Which of the following are goals of treatment for anorexia nervosa? Select all that apply.

   _____ Reinstitution of normal nutrition or reversal of the severe state of malnutrition

   _____ Resolution of disturbed patterns of family interaction

   _____ Individual psychotherapy to correct deficits and distortions of psychologic functioning

   _____ Neurologic assessment to evaluate for physical therapy

2. What is the purpose of developing a behavioral contract with the anorexia nervosa patient? Select all that apply.

_____ Allow the patient to have some individual control and responsibility for the contract

_____ Gradually reverse the malnutrition

_____ Get the weight back to normal quickly

_____ Establish a structured program with periods of observation around meals to ensure compliance

Exercise 2

 Virtual Hospital Activity

 30 minutes

Note: For this exercise, you will need to observe and consider four video interactions in two different periods of care before answering questions. Therefore you may want to read questions 1 through 6 first and then take notes while you view the videos.

- Sign in to work at Pacific View Regional Hospital for Period of Care 2. (*Note:* If you are already in the virtual hospital from a previous exercise, click on **Leave the Floor** and then **Restart the Program** to get to the sign-in window.)
- From the Patient List, select Tiffany Sheldon (Room 305).
- Click on **Go to Nurses' Station**.
- Click on **305** at the bottom of the screen to go to Tiffany Sheldon's room.
- Click on **Patient Care** and then on **Nurse-Client Interactions**.
- Select and view the videos titled **1115: Managing Anorexia Nervosa** and **1130: Monitoring Compliance**. (*Note:* Check the virtual clock to see whether enough time has elapsed. You can use the fast-forward feature to advance the time by 2-minute intervals if the video is not yet available. Then click again on **Patient Care** and **Nurse-Client Interactions** to refresh the screen.)
- When you have finished viewing these videos, click on **Leave the Floor**.
- At the Floor Menu, select **Restart the Program**.
- Sign in again, this time for Period of Care 3, and select Tiffany Sheldon (Room 305).
- Click on **Go to Nurses' Station** and then on **305** at the bottom of your screen.
- Click on **Patient Care** and then on **Nurse-Client Interactions**.
- Select and view the videos titled **1500: Relapse—Contributing Factors** and **1530: Facilitating Success**. (*Note:* Check the virtual clock to see whether enough time has elapsed. You can use the fast-forward feature to advance the time by 2-minute intervals if the video is not yet available. Then click again on **Patient Care** and **Nurse-Client Interactions** to refresh the screen.)
- Watch these interactions and then complete questions 1 through 6.

1. List four items that Tiffany has agreed to in her eating contract.

2. What statement does Tiffany Sheldon make during the video interactions that may lead you to believe she has concerns about her weight (disordered eating) and caloric intake?

3. What possible rationale might the nurse have for asking Tiffany Sheldon's mother whether she (the nurse) could speak to the adolescent alone?

4. What behavioral modification plans are implemented and discussed with Tiffany Sheldon? What are these plans specifically designed to monitor?

5. What purpose would monitoring Tiffany Sheldon in the bathroom serve in regard to food intake?

6. What is refeeding syndrome? (*Hint:* See Complications of Eating Disorders in Chapter 21 in the textbook.)

7. Based on the available information, is Tiffany Sheldon at risk for developing refeeding syndrome? State your rationale.

8. List at least two assessments that could lead to early identification of refeeding syndrome. (*Hint:* See Box 34-3 in the textbook.)

For questions 9 through 14, indicate whether each statement is true or false. If a statement is false, provide a rationale.

9. _____ The use of the behavioral contract has been consistently successful in the treatment program for anorexia nervosa. (True/False)

10. _____ The self-damaging behaviors of anorexia nervosa are a result of the patient's distorted body image and self-awareness, as well as feelings of self-doubt, ineffectiveness, helplessness, and lack of control. (True/False)

11. _____ Individual team members can make alterations to the behavior modification plan based on their individual interactions with the patient. (True/False)

12. _____ If the patient views the behavioral plan as coercive and becomes depressed by the approach, it is possible that weight gain may not be sustained outside of the hospital. (True/False)

13. _____ Family therapy needs to be directed toward disengagement and redirection of malfunctioning processes in the family. (True/False)

14. _____ Prevention of anorexia nervosa is very straightforward and usually very effective. (True/False)

LESSON 14

Nursing Care of the Child with Anorexia Nervosa

Reading Assignment: Behavioral Health Problems of Adolescence (Chapter 21)

Patient: Tiffany Sheldon, Room 305

Objectives:

1. Perform a nutritional assessment of the adolescent with anorexia nervosa.
2. Discuss the special care needs of the adolescent with anorexia nervosa.
3. Identify the contents and goal of the behavioral or "eating" contract.
4. Describe the psychologic implications of food intake in relation to perceived body image in the adolescent with anorexia nervosa.

Exercise 1

Virtual Hospital Activity

20 minutes

- Sign in to work at Pacific View Regional Hospital for Period of Care 2. (*Note:* If you are already in the virtual hospital from a previous exercise, click on **Leave the Floor** and then **Restart the Program** to get to the sign-in window.)
- From the Patient List, select Tiffany Sheldon (Room 305).
- Click on **Go to Nurses' Station**.
- Click on **Chart** and then on **305**.
- Click on **Consultations** and review the Nutrition Consult at 1115.
- Click on **Return to Nurses' Station** and then on **305** at the bottom of your screen to go to Tiffany Sheldon's room.
- Click on **Patient Care** and then on **Nurse-Client Interactions**.
- Select and view the videos titled **1115: Managing Anorexia Nervosa** and **1130: Monitoring Compliance**. (*Note:* Check the virtual clock to see whether enough time has elapsed. You can use the fast-forward feature to advance the time by 2-minute intervals if the video is not yet available. Then click again on **Patient Care** and **Nurse-Client Interactions** to refresh the screen.)

1. The dietitian has been working with Tiffany Sheldon and is aware of her history. In the 1115 video interaction, what is the purpose of the visit with Tiffany Sheldon? Select all that apply.

   _____ To develop the eating contract

   _____ To get Tiffany Sheldon's agreement about the eating contract

   _____ To assess Tiffany Sheldon's current nutritional status

   _____ To present Tiffany Sheldon with a menu to help in selection of a diet

2. What concern does Tiffany Sheldon express during the video interaction with the dietitian?
   a. She is concerned about when she will be discharged from the hospital.
   b. She is concerned that she will not be able to consume all the calories in the contract.
   c. She is concerned that the diet will make her more constipated.
   d. She is concerned that the diet will make her gain weight too quickly.

3. What would be a reasonable weight-gain goal for Tiffany Sheldon?

4. Because one of the signs of congestive heart failure (CHF) is weight gain, how would you determine that Tiffany Sheldon's weight gain is *not* a result of CHF?

5. What are possible barriers to Tiffany Sheldon being successful in negotiating the eating contract?
   a. Difficulty thinking clearly as a result of her poor nutritional status
   b. Inability to find hospital foods that are acceptable to her
   c. Unwillingness to remain in the hospital
   d. Concern about missing school

6. The dietitian is working with a treatment team to help monitor progress. What is the most important medical risk involved in developing a nutritional plan for Tiffany Sheldon?
   a. Possible physical injury from too much exercise
   b. Worsening constipation from increasing the diet
   c. Complications of refeeding syndrome, leading to severe metabolic abnormalities and cardiac complications

7. What is the value of establishing a "maintenance weight range"?
   a. Helps the patient to feel some control
   b. Encourages healthy dietary habits
   c. Teaches the patient that uncontrollable weight gain is not inevitable
   d. All of the above

8. The expected outcome of the behavioral contract is to ensure that expectations are met consistently. To promote this outcome, which of the following are important elements? Select all that apply.

_____ All team members agree with the plan

_____ All team members understand the plan

_____ There is a continuity of caregivers (team members)

_____ Team members communicate clearly to avoid communicating misunderstanding to the patient

_____ Consult with the patient regarding progress

_____ Provide the patient with positive feedback for accomplishments

→ • Click on **Leave the Floor** and then **Restart the Program**.
 • Sign in for Period of Care 3 and select Tiffany Sheldon (Room 305).
 • Click on **Go to Nurses' Station**.
 • Click on **Chart** and then on **305** for Tiffany Sheldon's chart.
 • Click on **Consultations** and review the Psychiatric Consult at 1500 on Wednesday.

9. The main goals of psychotherapy in the adolescent with anorexia nervosa are which of the following? Select all that apply.

_____ To promote the correction of metabolic abnormalities

_____ To support the eating contract and help patient understand the illness

_____ To form a therapeutic alliance that permits open discussion of the patient's feelings and helps develop more appropriate ways to communicate and cope

_____ To provide individual cognitive therapy to deal with environmental, familial, and personal conditions that may lead to anorexia nervosa

10. Identify three underlying issues that the psychiatrist identifies as contributing factors in Tiffany Sheldon's illness.

For questions 11 through 14, indicate whether each statement is true or false. If a statement is false, provide a rationale.

11. _____ An additional purpose for psychotherapy in anorexia nervosa is to help the patient develop a locus of control in order to express herself in acceptable ways. (True/False)

12. _____ Daily exercise is an important part of the anorexia nervosa recovery plan and a way for the patient to relieve stress. (True/False)

13. _____ It is important for the patient to understand that the team is in control of the contract and that the patient must obey all parts of the contract without question. (True/False)

14. _____ It is important to provide family members with support to help them deal with the pressures of managing a patient with anorexia nervosa. (True/False)

LESSON **15**

Emergent Nursing Care of the Child with Meningitis

🔖 **Reading Assignment:** Communication and Physical Assessment of the Child
(Chapter 6)
The Child with Cerebral Dysfunction (Chapter 37)

Patient: Stephanie Brown, Room 304

Objectives:

1. Differentiate between bacterial and aseptic meningitis.
2. Perform a neurologic assessment on a child who is diagnosed with meningitis.
3. Analyze laboratory findings associated with childhood meningitis.
4. Describe the pathophysiology of meningitis.
5. Participate in the care of the child with meningitis.

Exercise 1

✏️ **Writing Activity**

 15 minutes

1. Match each of the following terms or phrases with its correct definition or description.

Term/Phrase	Definition/Description
_____ Meningitis	a. Viral inflammation of the meninges
_____ Mode of meningitis transmission	b. Greatest morbidity between birth and 4 years
_____ Bacterial meningitis	c. Vascular dissemination of mucosal organisms frequently from the nasopharyngeal site
_____ Predisposition to meningitis	d. Pyogenic inflammation of the meninges
_____ Aseptic meningitis	e. Inflammation of the membranes covering the brain and spinal cord

2. What are common clinical manifestations of meningitis in children and adolescents?

Exercise 2

 Virtual Hospital Activity

 45 minutes

- Sign in to work at Pacific View Regional Hospital for Period of Care 1. (*Note:* If you are already in the virtual hospital from a previous exercise, click on **Leave the Floor** and then **Restart the Program** to get to the sign-in window.)
- From the Patient List, select Stephanie Brown (Room 304).
- Click on **Go to Nurses' Station**.
- Click on **304** at the bottom of your screen to go to Stephanie Brown's room.
- Click on **Patient Care**.
- Click on **Physical Assessment**.
- Click on **Head & Neck**.
- Click on **Neurologic** and view the assessment.

 1. Identify the physiologic basis for Stephanie Brown's headache. (*Hint:* See the section on Bacterial Meningitis: Clinical Manifestations in Chapter 37 of your textbook.)

 - Click on **Chart**.
- Click on **304** to view Stephanie Brown's chart.
- Click on **Emergency Department** and review.
- Click on and read the **Nurse's Notes** and **Physician's Notes**.

2. List the clinical manifestations of meningitis exhibited by Stephanie Brown in the Emergency Department.

• Click on **Chart** and then click on **304**.

• Click on and read the **History and Physical** section of Stephanie Brown's chart.

3. Describe the standard Glasgow Coma Scale (GCS) and list the three-part assessment of the coma scale. Then explain how the pediatric version of the GCS differs in assessment.

 • Click on **Laboratory Reports**. Review the findings recorded in the Emergency Department on Monday at 0100.

 4. Below, list the abnormal laboratory findings you noted for Stephanie Brown in the Laboratory Reports. For each abnormal finding, give the normal range of results. Finally, what does each finding indicate? (*Hint:* Common laboratory tests are outlined in Appendix C of the textbook).

Laboratory Test	Results	Normal Range	Indications

• Now click on **Diagnostic Reports** and review the summary of Stephanie Brown's lumbar puncture.

5. When a child has suspected meningitis, spinal fluid pressure can be measured during the lumbar puncture with a manometer. What is Stephanie Brown's spinal fluid pressure? The normal range for a child her age is 60-100 mm H_2O. What is the significance of these results in relation to Stephanie Brown's condition?

 6. Below, list the cerebral spinal fluid (CSF) results from Stephanie Brown's lumbar puncture on Monday. For each finding, give the normal range of results and identify what each of Stephanie Brown's findings indicates. (*Hint:* Common laboratory tests are outlined in Appendix C of the textbook.)

CSF (Lumbar)	Results	Normal Range	Indications

7. What is the rationale for placing Stephanie Brown in respiratory isolation?

 • Click on **Physician's Orders** and review.

8. What medication is ordered for Stephanie Brown for a high temperature?

9. Based on Stephanie Brown's status on admission to the Emergency Department, prioritize the following nursing interventions by numbering them from 1 to 7 (with 1 being the highest priority and 7 the lowest). In this case, Stephanie Brown has just had diagnostic studies completed in the Emergency Department. Her vital signs and neurologic signs were taken 30 minutes ago.

_____ Elevating Stephanie Brown's head of bed 45 degrees

_____ Monitoring neurologic signs hourly

_____ Administering vancomycin 180 mg IV over 1 hour

_____ Placing Stephanie Brown in contact and respiratory isolation

_____ Inserting a peripheral IV and administering a normal saline bolus of 20 mL/kg over 20 minutes

_____ Monitoring Stephanie Brown's vital signs hourly

_____ Implementing seizure precautions

10. What is the rationale for having the head of Stephanie Brown's bed elevated 45 degrees?

11. Describe the standard isolation technique for the child with meningitis in an acute care center. (*Note:* You may describe the standard practice in an institution where you work as staff member or student.)

12. What is the physiologic basis for giving Stephanie Brown a normal saline bolus in the Emergency Department? (*Hint:* See the Systems Review section of the Emergency Department record in the chart.)

• Click on the **Return to Room 304**.

• Click on **MAR** and review Stephanie Brown's records.

13. In nursing care of the child with suspected meningitis, what is a major priority regarding the administration of the first dose of antibiotics.

Now let's go to the Medication Room and prepare to administer all of the 0730 and 0800 medications ordered for Stephanie Brown.

• First, click on **Return to Room 304**.

• Click on the **Medication Room**.

• Click on **MAR** to determine what medications Stephanie Brown should receive for 0730 and 0800. You may review the MAR at any time to verify the correct medication order. (*Hint:* Remember to look at the patient name on the MAR to make sure you have the correct record—you must click on the tab with Stephanie Brown's room number within the MAR.) Click on **Return to Medication Room** after reviewing the correct MAR.

• Click on **Unit Dosage** and then on drawer **304**.

• Select the medications you would like to administer. For each medication you select, click on **Put Medication on Tray**. When you are finished, click on **Close Drawer**.

• Click on **View Medication Room**.

• Now click on **Automated System** and **Login**.

• Select the correct patient and drawer according to the medication you want to administer. (*Hint:* This automated system is for controlled substances only.) Then click on **Open Drawer**.

• Select the medication you would like to administer, click on **Put Medication on Tray**, and then click on **Close Drawer**.

• Click on **View Medication Room**.

• Click on **Preparation** and select the medication to administer.

• Click on **Prepare** and wait for the Preparation Wizard to appear. Select the medication you would like to administer, click on **Prepare**, follow the prompts, and then click on **Next**.

• Choose the correct patient and then click on **Finish**.

• Repeat the previous three steps until all medications that you want to administer are prepared.

• You can click on **Review Your Medications** and then click on **Return to Medication Room** when ready. When back in the Medication Room, go directly to Stephanie Brown's room by clicking on **304** at the bottom of the screen.

• In Stephanie Brown's room, administer the medications, utilizing the six rights of medication administration.

• After you have collected the appropriate assessment data and are ready for administration, click on **Patient Care** and then on **Medication Administration**.

• Verify that the correct patient and medication(s) appear in the left-hand window.

• Highlight the medication you wish to administer; then click the down arrow next to Select. From the drop-down menu, select **Administer** and complete the Administration Wizard by providing any information requested.

• When the Wizard stops asking for information, click on **Administer to Patient**.

- Specify **Yes** when asked whether this administration should be recorded in the MAR. Finally, click **Finish**.
- Complete these steps for each medication you wish to administer.

14. In the mock MAR form below, document the medications you administered.

Medication Administration Record

Medication/Dose	2300-0700	0700-1500	1500-2300

 15. Stephanie Brown is receiving maintenance IV fluids with strict intake and output to prevent what severe complication? (*Hint:* See the discussion of Nutrition and Hydration in Chapter 37 of your textbook.)

 16. List three physical signs and three behavioral/personality signs in a child Stephanie Brown's age that the nurse should recognize as manifestations of the condition identified in question 15. (*Hint:* See Box 37-1 in your textbook.)

• To answer questions 17 through 19, you will need to consult the Drug Guide located in the bottom left-hand corner of your screen.

• To access the Drug Guide, click on the **Drug** icon. When the Drug Guide opens, use the Search box or scroll through the list of drugs at the top of the screen; select **vancomycin**.

17. Provide the rationale for the IV administration of this drug (versus oral administration).

18. Briefly describe the procedure for administering vancomycin intravenously to a child Stephanie Brown's age. Include directions for reconstitution and length and method of administration.

19. List three serious side effects for which the nurse should be vigilant during and after the administration of this medication.

Now let's see how you did administering Stephanie Brown's medications.

 • Click on **Return to Room 304**.

• Click on **Leave the Floor** at the bottom of your screen. From the Floor Menu, select **Look at Your Preceptor's Evaluation**. Then click on **Medication Scorecard**.

• Review the scorecard to see whether or not you correctly administered the appropriate medication(s). If not, why do you think you were incorrect? According to Table C in this scorecard, what resources should be used and what important assessments should be completed before administering the medication(s)? Did you use these resources and perform these assessments correctly?

• Print a copy of the Medication Scorecard for your instructor to evaluate.

Nursing Care of the Hospitalized Child

 Reading Assignment: Perspectives of Pediatric Nursing (Chapter 1)
The Child with Cerebral Dysfunction (Chapter 37)

Patient: Stephanie Brown, Room 304

Objectives:

1. Describe the purpose of the nursing process in patient care.
2. Develop a plan of care for a hospitalized child with bacterial meningitis.

Exercise 1

 Writing Activity

15 minutes

1. Define the nursing process.

2. What are the five steps of the nursing process?

   (1)

   (2)

   (3)

   (4)

   (5)

3. Describe the actions taken in each of the steps of the nursing process.

(1)

(2)

(3)

(4)

(5)

Exercise 2

  Virtual Hospital Activity

 45 minutes

- Sign in to work at Pacific View Regional Hospital for Period of Care 3. (*Note:* If you are already in the virtual hospital from a previous exercise, click on **Leave the Floor** and then **Restart the Program** to get to the sign-in window.)
- From the Patient List, select Stephanie Brown (Room 304).
- Click on **Go to Nurses' Station** and then on **Chart**.
- Click on **304** to view Stephanie Brown's chart.
- Click on and review the **History and Physical** and **Nursing Admission** sections of the chart.
- Click on **Nurse's Notes** and review the notes for Monday starting at 0600. The plan of care will begin with Stephanie Brown's admission to the Pediatrics Unit.
- Click on **Physician's Notes** and review the information given.
- Review Lesson 15 in this workbook.

Use the following steps to complete the tables in questions 1 through 3. (*Hint:* It may be helpful to refer to the Bacterial Meningitis: Nursing Care Management section in Chapter 37 of your textbook to complete these questions.)

- Identify three nursing diagnoses* for Stephanie Brown and record these in column 1 of each of the three tables.
- Identify subjective/objective data or risk factors from Stephanie Brown's assessment data that support each nursing diagnosis. Record this information in column 2 of each table.
- Supply an outcome for each nursing diagnosis (column 3 of each table).
- List three priority nursing interventions for Stephanie Brown in relation to each nursing diagnosis (column 4 of each table).
- Supply rationales for the nursing interventions in column 5 of each table.

Note: This nursing care plan is just one prototype and the nursing diagnoses used in the answer key are examples. You may develop other acceptable nursing care plans and nursing diagnoses to meet your institution's requirements.

1. Complete the table below for your first nursing diagnosis.

Nursing Diagnosis	Support for Diagnosis	Outcome	Nursing Interventions	Rationale

2. Complete the table below for your second nursing diagnosis.

Nursing Diagnosis	Support for Diagnosis	Outcome	Nursing Interventions	Rationale

3. Complete the table below for your third nursing diagnosis.

Nursing Diagnosis	Support for Diagnosis	Outcome	Nursing Interventions	Rationale

4. Although evaluation is listed as the last step in the nursing process, it is imperative that this process begin during assessment and continue until the patient is discharged home. List the four key evaluation criteria outlined in Chapter 1 in the textbook.

LESSON 17

Nursing Care of the Hospitalized Child with Bacterial Meningitis

Reading Assignment: Communication and Physical Assessment of the Child (Chapter 6)
Pain Assessment and Management in Children (Chapter 7)
The Child with Cerebral Dysfunction (Chapter 37)
The Child with Neuromuscular or Muscular Dysfunction (Chapter 40)

Patient: Stephanie Brown, Room 304

Objectives:

1. Perform a neurologic assessment on a child who is diagnosed with meningitis.
2. Participate in the care of the child with meningitis.

Exercise 1

 Virtual Hospital Activity

 45 minutes

- Sign in to work at Pacific View Regional Hospital for Period of Care 2. (*Note:* If you are already in the virtual hospital from a previous exercise, click on **Leave the Floor** and then **Restart the Program** to get to the sign-in window.)
- From the Patient List, select Stephanie Brown (Room 304).
- Click on **Go to Nurses' Station**.
- Click on **Chart** and then on **304**.
- Click on **Emergency Department** and review the report.
- Click on and review the **Physician's Orders** and **Physician's Notes** for Wednesday at 0900.
- Click on **Return to Nurses' Station**.
- Click on **304** at the bottom of the screen to go to Stephanie Brown's room.
- Click on **Patient Care** and then on **Nurse-Client Interactions**.
- Select and view the video titled **1120: Preventing Spread of Disease**. (*Note:* Check the virtual clock to see whether enough time has elapsed. You can use the fast-forward feature to advance the time by 2-minute intervals if the video is not yet available. Then click again on **Patient Care** and **Nurse-Client Interactions** to refresh the screen.)

1. What might explain why the physician decreased Stephanie Brown's IV rate to 10 mL/hr?

2. How did Stephanie Brown's nurse explain the basis for the respiratory isolation?

3. Based on your earlier review of the Physician's Notes, what was the physician's most likely rationale for discontinuing the respiratory isolation and vancomycin for Stephanie Brown?

➤ • Now select and view the video titled **1145: Teaching—Disease Sequelae**. (*Note:* Check the virtual clock to see whether enough time has elapsed. You can use the fast-forward feature to advance the time by 2-minute intervals if the video is not yet available. Then click again on **Patient Care** and **Nurse-Client Interactions** to refresh the screen.)

You may also want to refer to the Reflexes section in Chapter 6 and the Bacterial Meningitis: Clinical Manifestations section in Chapter 37 of your textbook.

4. Describe the significance of the Kernig and Brudzinski signs and how each sign is elicited.

5. What causes nuchal rigidity? What is the significance of this finding in a child with meningitis?

6. Compare Stephanie Brown's Kernig sign, Brudzinski sign, and the nuchal rigidity results described in the Emergency Department Physician's Progress note on Tuesday with the description in the Physician's Progress note on Wednesday 0900.

 • Click on **Chart** and then on **304**.
   • Click on **Consultations** and review the Audiology Consult.

 Review the Auditory Testing section (including Table 6-10) in Chapter 6 of your textbook.

 7. Explain the basis for obtaining the audiogram in Stephanie Brown. What are the results of the audiogram? How soon after recovery from meningitis is the audiogram usually repeated? (*Hint:* See the sections Bacterial Meningitis: Drugs and Bacterial Meningitis: Prognosis in Chapter 37 of your textbook.)

 • Click on **Return to Room 304**.
   • Click on **Clinical Alerts** and review.

8. What does the Clinical Alert say regarding Stephanie Brown's abdominal assessment?

9. When did Stephanie Brown have her last bowel movement?

 • Click on **Chart** and then on **304**.
• Review the **Physician's Orders** for 1100 on Wednesday.

10. What medication is ordered for Stephanie Brown at this time?

 • Click on **Return to Room 304**.
• Click on the **Drug** icon in the lower left corner of your screen.

11. Using the Drug Guide, complete the following table for the drug you identified in the previous question. Relate your answers specifically to Stephanie Brown's need for the medication.

Name of Medication	Classification	Action	Dosage	Frequency	Route

 • Click on **Return to Room 304**.
• Click on **Medication Room**.
• Prepare the medication you identified in question 10.
• When you have finished the steps of the Preparation Wizard, click on **Return to Medication Room** and then on **304** to go to Stephanie Brown's room.
• Administer the medication, using the six rights of medication administration.
• After you have collected the appropriate assessment data and are ready for administration, click on **Patient Care** and then on **Medication Administration**.
• Verify that the correct patient and medication(s) appear in the left-hand window. Then click the down arrow next to Select. From the drop-down menu, select **Administer** and complete the Administration Wizard by providing any information requested.
• When the Wizard stops asking for information, click **Administer to Patient**.
• Specify **Yes** when asked whether this administration should be recorded in the MAR.
• Finally, click **Finish**.

12. In the mock MAR form below, document the medication you just administered to Stephanie Brown. Indicate the time you gave it in the correct column.

Medication Administration Record

Medication/Dose	2300-0700	0700-1500	1500-2300

Now let's see how you did!

- Click on **Leave the Floor** at the bottom of your screen. From the Floor Menu, select **Look at Your Preceptor's Evaluation**. Then click on **Medication Scorecard**.
- Review the scorecard to see whether or not you correctly administered the appropriate medication. If not, why do you think you were incorrect? According to Table C in this scorecard, what resources should be used and what important assessments should be completed before administering the medication(s)? Did you use these resources and perform these assessments correctly?
- Print a copy of the Medication Scorecard for your instructor to evaluate.

 Review Table 7-2 and the Pain Intensity section of Chapter 7 of your textbook.

- Click on **Return to Menu**.
- Click on **Restart the Program**.
- Sign in for Period of Care 2 and select Stephanie Brown (Room 304) as the patient.
- Click on **Go to Nurses' Station**.
- Click on **EPR** and then on **Login**.
- Select **304** from the Patient drop-down menu and **Vital Signs** from the Category drop-down menu.

13. Compare Stephanie Brown's blood pressure and pain-scale rating on Wednesday 0700 with her blood pressure and pain-scale rating on Wednesday at 1100.

Use the FACES pain rating scale below to answer questions 14 and 15.

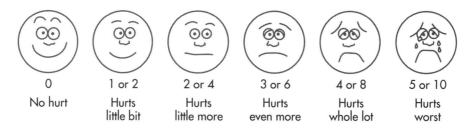

| 0 | 1 or 2 | 2 or 4 | 3 or 6 | 4 or 8 | 5 or 10 |
| No hurt | Hurts little bit | Hurts little more | Hurts even more | Hurts whole lot | Hurts worst |

14. Identify the face that matches Stephanie Brown's description of her headache recorded on Wednesday at 1100.

15. Identify the three scales used in the FACES system.

→ • Click on **Exit EPR**.
  • Click on **Chart** and then on **304**.
  • Once again, review the **Physician's Orders** for Stephanie Brown.

16. What is ordered that can be administered to alleviate her headache?

→ • Click on **Return to Nurses' Station**.
  • Now click on the **Drug** icon in the lower left corner of your screen.

17. Using the Drug Guide as your reference, complete the following table for the medication you identified in the previous question.

Name of Medication	Classification	Action	Dosage	Frequency	Route

• Click on **Return to Nurses' Station**.
 • Click on **Chart** and then on **304**.
 • Review the **Nurse's Notes** for Tuesday at 2300 and Wednesday at 0600.

18. Based on your assessment of Stephanie Brown at this time, what route would be appropriate for administering the medication you identified in question 15? State your rationale for choosing this route.

 19. Briefly describe the indication(s) for administering baclofen to a child with cerebral palsy. (*Hint:* Use the Drug Guide and see Chapter 40 in your textbook.)

LESSON 18

Nursing Care of the Hospitalized Child with Cerebral Palsy

Reading Assignment: Pain Assessment and Management in Children (Chapter 7)
The Child with Gastrointestinal Dysfunction (Chapter 33)
The Child with Neuromuscular or Muscular Dysfunction
(Chapter 40)

Patient: Stephanie Brown, Room 304

Objectives:

1. Participate in the care of the child with cerebral palsy.
2. Discuss the special needs of a child with cerebral palsy.
3. Identify measures to decrease anxiety in a child and family with cerebral palsy.

Exercise 1

Virtual Hospital Activity

50 minutes

- Sign in to work at Pacific View Regional Hospital for Period of Care 3. (*Note:* If you are already in the virtual hospital from a previous exercise, click on **Leave the Floor** and then **Restart the Program** to get to the sign-in window.)
- From the Patient List, select Stephanie Brown (Room 304).
- Click on **Go to Nurses' Station**.
- Click on **304** at the bottom of the screen to go to the patient's room.
- Click on **Patient Care** and then on **Nurse-Client Interactions**.
- Select and view the video titled **1500: Assessment—IV Site**. (*Note:* Check the virtual clock to see whether enough time has elapsed. You can use the fast-forward feature to advance the time by 2-minute intervals if the video is not yet available. Then click again on **Patient Care** and **Nurse-Client Interactions** to refresh the screen.)

  1. How did the nurse describe the IV site in the video? What are the implications of her findings?

135

• Now select and view the video titled **1510: Nurse-Patient Communication**. (*Note:* Check the virtual clock to see whether enough time has elapsed. You can use the fast-forward feature to advance the time by 2-minute intervals if the video is not yet available. Then click again on **Patient Care** and **Nurse-Client Interactions** to refresh the screen.)

2. Describe the purpose of applying EMLA cream prior to restarting the IV as stated by the nurse in the video.

Let's take a virtual leap in time to see whether the EMLA cream was applied.

 • Click on **Leave the Floor** and then **Restart the Program**.
• Sign in for Period of Care 4. (*Remember:* You are not able to visit patients or administer medications during Period of Care 4. You are able to review patient records only.)
• Click on **MAR** and then on tab **304**.
• Review Stephanie Brown's MAR for Wednesday at 1900.

3. At what time was the EMLA cream administered? Why should the nurse wait 60 minutes after EMLA is applied to the skin before the IV is restarted?

 4. List three alternative topical analgesics that may be used for a child Stephanie Brown's age if EMLA is unavailable or if length of time is a factor in the insertion of a peripheral IV (*Hint:* See the section on Transmucosal and Transdermal Analgesia in Chapter 7 in your textbook.)

Now, let's return to Period of Care 3 to continue your care for Stephanie Brown.

 • Click on **Return to Nurses' Station**.
• Once again, click on **Leave the Floor** and **Restart the Program**.
• Sign in for Period of Care 3 and select Stephanie Brown (Room 304).
• Click on **Go to Nurses' Station**.
• Click on **Chart** and then on **304**.
• Click on **History and Physical** and review.
• Click on **Nursing Admissions** and review.

5. List the predisposing maternal and perinatal factors in Stephanie Brown's history that may have contributed to the development of cerebral palsy.

 • Click on **Consultations** and read the PT/OT Consult.

6. State the findings of the PT/OT Consult.

7. What specific therapy is recommended for Stephanie Brown by the physical therapist based on the findings during the consult?

8. What is an ankle-foot orthosis (AFO)? When did Stephanie Brown start wearing an AFO? State the purpose of the AFO. (*Hint:* See Therapeutic Management: General Concepts and Therapeutic Management: Therapies, Education, Recreation for cerebral palsy in Chapter 40 in your textbook.)

 • Click on **Nurse's Notes**.
   • Review the Nurse's Notes from the Emergency Department admission through Wednesday.

9. What specific request does Stephanie Brown's mother make of the social worker? (*Hint:* Read the note on Tuesday at 1500.)

10. Describe activities that can help Stephanie Brown's mother cope with the anxiety associated with her child's hospitalization and life-threatening illness.

11. Describe age-appropriate activities that can help Stephanie Brown cope with the anxiety associated with hospitalization and respiratory isolation.

12. What recommendations could you give Stephanie Brown's mother to promote her daughter's daily bowel movement? (*Hint:* See Constipation in Chapter 33 of your textbook.)

→ • Click on **Return to Nurses' Station**.
  • Click on **304** at the bottom of the screen to go to Stephanie Brown's room.
  • Click on **Patient Care** and then on **Nurse-Client Interactions**.
  • Select and view the video titled **1530: Preventive Measures**. (*Note:* Check the virtual clock to see whether enough time has elapsed. You can use the fast-forward feature to advance the time by 2-minute intervals if the video is not yet available. Then click again on **Patient Care** and **Nurse-Client Interactions** to refresh the screen.)

13. What specific recommendation does the physical therapist make to Stephanie Brown's mother on the consult note and during the video?

Developing an EBP Summary Review: Meningitis in Children— Effectiveness of Vaccines

Reading Assignment: The Child with Cerebral Dysfunction (Chapter 37)

Patient: Stephanie Brown, Room 304

Objectives:

1. Develop an EBP summary review of the effectiveness of vaccines for meningitis in children.

Before beginning this lesson, complete Lessons 15 through 18. These lessons focus on Stephanie Brown, who was admitted to the hospital because of suspected meningitis. Lessons 15 through 18 gave you an overview of the care required for a patient possibly experiencing meningitis. This lesson gives you an opportunity to explore the evidence on preventive vaccinations for children with bacterial meningitis.

Exercise 1

Writing Activity

60 minutes

Before you begin developing your EBP summary review, remember the following guidelines:

- Begin by establishing the purpose of the review.
- Next, think about the key terms or words you will use to search the literature.
- Once you decide on your search terms, think about where you will search.
- What organizations might have websites that provide information on this subject?
- What national agencies might have studies that review the information? (Remember to search on the Cochrane Collaboration and AHRQ websites.)
- Remember to search both nursing and medical literature.
- Once your search is completed, critically review each article and evaluate the evidence. In a sentence or two, summarize the study. Include the study purpose, sample, design, procedures, and findings.

- Apply the findings to nursing practice. What recommendations can you make to clinical practice?
- In the final box of the EBP summary review, include all the references you used in the summary. Be sure you write these in an appropriate reference style for your nursing program.

1. Using the guidelines just summarized, complete the following EBP summary review of the effectiveness of preventive vaccines for bacterial meningitis in children.

Ask the Question

Question

Search the Evidence	**List at least three search engines or websites you used to obtain information.**
Databases Searched	
Search Strategies	

Critically Analyze the Evidence

Provide a concise synopsis of each article relevant to the subject.

Summary of Findings

Apply Evidence Recommendations

What nursing implications can be recommended based on your summary of the findings? Describe below.

References   **List at least four references you used in your review.**

LESSON **20**

Care of the Infant with Respiratory Distress

 Reading Assignment: Health Problems During Infancy (Chapter 13)

Family-Centered Care of the Child During Illness and
Hospitalization (Chapter 26)

The Child with Disturbance of Oxygen and Carbon Dioxide
Exchange (Chapter 31)

The Child with Respiratory Dysfunction (Chapter 32)

Patient: Carrie Richards, Room 303

Objectives:

1. Recognize signs of acute respiratory distress in an infant.
2. Describe the nursing care of an infant with respiratory syncytial virus (RSV)/bronchiolitis.

Exercise 1

Writing Activity

30 minutes

1. What is RSV? Briefly describe the characteristic progression of this illness in children. Also
   identify any associated clinical manifestations.

2. How is this illness transmitted?

3. Describe the steps that can be taken to reduce or prevent the transmission of this illness.

4. List four priority nursing interventions for an infant with RSV.

5. What medication may be given as a prophylactic treatment?

6. Who should receive the medication, and when should this medication be administered?

7. When should this medication be administered (time of year)? How is this medication administered (route)?

Exercise 2

 Virtual Hospital Activity

 50 minutes

- Sign in to work at Pacific View Regional Hospital for Period of Care 1. (*Note:* If you are already in the virtual hospital from a previous exercise, click on **Leave the Floor** and then **Restart the Program** to get to the sign-in window.)
- From the Patient List, select Carrie Richards (Room 303).
- Click on **Go to Nurses' Station**.
- Click on **Chart** and then on **303** for Carrie Richards' chart.
- Click on **Emergency Department** and review this record.

1. What are Carrie Richards' vital signs on admission to the Emergency Department at 1630? Place an asterisk (*) after any finding that is out of the normal range for a child her age.

2. Briefly describe the findings recorded for Carrie Richards in the Systems Review portion of the Emergency Department Record and in the Emergency Department Nurse's Note at 1800. Place an asterisk (*) after any finding that is out of the normal range for a child her age.

3. List the five cardinal clinical signs of respiratory distress in an infant. Place an asterisk (*) after any sign demonstrated by Carrie Richards on admission to the Emergency Department.

→ • Still in the Emergency Department section of the chart, compare the findings in the Emergency Department Nurse's Notes at 1800 and 1900.

4. What clinical signs documented by the nurse indicate a change in Carrie Richards' respiratory status at 1900?

5. What specific intervention is performed to improve Carrie Richards' oxygenation status?

6. What medication is administered to Carrie Richards to improve her respiratory status in the Emergency Department?

7. Describe the intended effect of this medication in a child with bronchiolitis/RSV who is wheezing and has a lower airway infection.

8. Describe how this medication is administered in an infant Carrie Richards' age. What is the rationale for this method of administration?

9. List at least two side effects of this medication.

10. Identify priority assessments that need to be performed after the nebulizer treatment is given.

11. What is the primary medical diagnosis listed for Carrie Richards?

12. List two nursing diagnoses for Carrie Richards based on your review of her status in the Emergency Department.

13. In the 1800 Emergency Department Nurse's Notes, an important clue is given in relation to the severity of Carrie Richards' status. What might lead you to conclude that her condition is poor? (*Hint:* Consider her age and developmental status.)

→ • Still in Carrie Richards chart, click on **Laboratory Reports**.

14. Below, fill in Carrie Richards' laboratory values recorded in the Emergency Department at 1800 on Tuesday. Place an asterisk (*) after any lab value that is out of the normal range for a child Carrie Richards' age. (*Hint:* See Appendix C, Common Laboratory Tests, in your textbook.)

Chemistry	Arterial Blood Gas
Glucose	pH
Sodium (serum)	PaO_2
Potassium	$PaCO_2$
Chloride	Oxygen sat
CO_2	
Creatinine	
BUN	
Calcium	

Urinalysis	Hematology
Color	WBC
Clarity	RBC
Glucose	Hgb
Bilirubin	Hct
Blood	Platelets
Spec gravity	Differential
pH	Segs
Protein	Bands
Ketones	Lymphocytes
WBC	Monocytes
	Eosinophils
	Basophils

→ • Click on **Emergency Department**. Once again, review the Emergency Department Nurse's
Notes for 1900 on Tuesday.

15. How is Carrie Richards' respiratory status described? What interventions other than the
nebulized medication administration and oxygen were performed to improve her respiratory
status? State the rationale for the intervention performed.

16. List the clinical signs, physical assessment findings, and any laboratory values that provide
a basis for determining Carrie Richards' hydration status on admission to the Emergency
Department.

17. Describe the intervention(s) used to hydrate Carrie Richards in the Emergency Department.

18. List two reasons Carrie Richards is not a candidate for oral hydration in the Emergency
Department.

19. Describe important assessment data that should be documented regarding Carrie Richards' IV site.

Care of the Hospitalized Infant

/OTD **Reading Assignment:** Communication and Physical Assessment of the Child
(Chapter 6)
Pediatric Variations of Nursing Interventions (Chapter 27)
Balance and Imbalance of Body Fluids (Chapter 28)
The Child with Respiratory Dysfunction (Chapter 32)

Patient: Carrie Richards, Room 303

Objectives:

1. Recognize signs of acute respiratory distress in an infant.
2. Describe the nursing care of an infant with respiratory syncytial virus (RSV)/bronchiolitis.
3. Participate in the care of an infant with respiratory distress.

Exercise 1

Virtual Hospital Activity

20 minutes

- Sign in to work at Pacific View Regional Hospital for Period of Care 1. (*Note:* If you are already in the virtual hospital from a previous exercise, click on **Leave the Floor** and then **Restart the Program** to get to the sign-in window.)
- From the Patient List, select Carrie Richards (Room 303).
- Click on **Get Report** and review.
- Click on **Go to Nurses' Station**.
- Click on **Chart** and then on **303**.
- Click on and review the **Emergency Department** record.
- Click on and review the **History and Physical**.
- Click on and review the **Nursing Admission** and the **Physician's Orders** for Tuesday 1700 and 2300.

1. Briefly summarize Carrie Richards' health history since birth.

2. Is Carrie Richards' immunization status current? If not, list the immunization(s) she should receive as soon as possible.

 • Before leaving the chart, record Carrie Richards' physical assessment findings on admission in the middle column of the table in question 3. (*Hint:* You can find these in the Emergency Department record.)
• Click on **Return to Nurses' Station**.
• Click on **303** at the bottom of the screen to go to Carrie Richards' room.
• Click on **Patient Care**.
• Click on **Physical Assessment**.
• Perform a focused assessment by selecting the various body areas (yellow buttons) and system subcategories (green buttons) as needed to complete question 3.

3. Record your findings from the physical assessment in the far-right column below. Then compare these current findings with those obtained on admission to the Emergency Department.

Findings	Admission 1700 Tuesday	Current Findings
Respiratory effort		
Breath sounds		
Adventitious lung sounds		
Sensory/activity level		
Capillary refill		
Pulses		
Supplemental oxygen		

• Still in Carrie Richards' room, click on **Nurse-Client Interactions**.
• Select and view the video titled **0730: Patient Assessment**. (*Note:* Check the virtual clock to see whether enough time has elapsed. You can use the fast-forward feature to advance the time by 2-minute intervals if the video is not yet available. Then click again on **Patient Care** and **Nurse-Client Interactions** to refresh the screen.)

4. How does the nurse assess Carrie Richards' respiratory status in the video?

5. Carrie Richards is 3½ months old. At this age, breathing is primarily:
   a. abdominal.
   b. diaphragmatic.

 • Click on **Take Vital Signs**.

6. Record Carrie Richards' vital sign results below.

Temperature

Heart rate

Respiratory rate

Oxygen saturation

Blood pressure

7. Based on Carrie Richards' current physical assessment findings and vital signs, what conclusion might be drawn about her respiratory status and general health at this time?

 • Click on **EPR** and **Login**.
   • Select **303** from the Patient drop-down menu.
   • Choose various categories as needed to record the vital signs and physical assessment findings you gathered in Carrie Richards' room. Be sure to include respiratory findings and IV status. (*Note:* The EPR may be printed for instructor evaluation.)

Exercise 2

 Virtual Hospital Activity

 45 minutes

   • Sign in to work at Pacific View Regional Hospital for Period of Care 3. (*Note:* If you are already in the virtual hospital from a previous exercise, click on **Leave the Floor** and then **Restart the Program** to get to the sign-in window.)
   • From the Patient List, select Carrie Richards (Room 303).

- Click on **Go to Nurses' Station**.
- Click on **Chart** and then on **303**.
- Click on and review the **Nurse's Notes**.
- Click on **Return to Nurses' Station**.
- Click on **EPR** and then **Login**.
- Select **303** from the Patient drop-down menu and **Respiratory** from the Category drop-down menu.

1. Summarize Carrie Richards' respiratory status at 1300 on Wednesday based on the 1240 Nurse's Notes and 1215 respiratory assessment data in the EPR.

→ • Still in the EPR, change the category to **Vital Signs**.

2. What is Carrie Richards' body temperature at 1445?

→ • Click on **Exit EPR**.
- Click on **MAR** and then on tab **303**.

3. What medication does Carrie Richards have ordered for fever or irritability?

Now let's go to the Medication Room and prepare to administer all of the 1500 medications ordered for Carrie Richards.

→ • First, click on **Return to Nurses' Station**.
- Next, click on **Medication Room**.
- Click on **MAR** to determine what medications Carrie Richards should receive at 1500. You may review the MAR at any time to verify the correct medication order. (*Hint:* Remember to look at the patient name on the MAR to make sure you have the correct record—you must click on the tab with Carrie Richards' room number within the MAR). Click on **Return to Medication Room** after reviewing the correct MAR.
- Click on **Unit Dosage** and then on drawer **303**.
- Select the medications you would like to administer. For each medication you select, click on **Put Medication on Tray**. When you are finished, click on **Close Drawer**.
- Click on **View Medication Room**.
- Now click on **Automated System** and **Login**.

- Select the correct patient and drawer according to the medication you want to administer. (*Hint:* This automated system is for controlled substances only.) Then click on **Open Drawer**.
- Select the medication you would like to administer, click on **Put Medication on Tray**, and then click on **Close Drawer**.
- Click on **View Medication Room** and then on **Preparation**. Select the medication to administer.
- Click on **Prepare** and wait for the Preparation Wizard to appear. If the Wizard requests information, provide your answer(s) and then click on **Next**.
- Choose the correct patient and then click on **Finish**.
- Repeat the previous three steps until all medications that you want to administer are prepared.
- You can click on **Review Your Medications** and then click on **Return to Medication Room** when ready. When back in the Medication Room, go directly to Carrie Richards' room by clicking on **303** at the bottom of the screen.
- In Carrie Richards' room, administer the medications, utilizing the six rights of medication administration.
- After you have collected the appropriate assessment data and are ready for administration, click on **Patient Care** and then on **Medication Administration**.
- Verify that the correct patient and medication(s) appear in the left-hand window. Then click the down arrow next to Select. From the drop-down menu, select **Administer** and complete the Administration Wizard by providing any information requested.
- When the Wizard stops asking for information, click on **Administer to Patient**.
- Specify **Yes** when asked whether this administration should be recorded in the MAR.
- Finally, click on **Finish**. Complete these steps for each medication you wish to administer.

Now let's see how you did!

- Click on **Leave the Floor** at the bottom of your screen.
- From the Floor Menu, select **Look at Your Preceptor's Evaluation**. Then click on **Medication Scorecard**.
- Review the scorecard to see whether or not you correctly administered the appropriate medication(s). If not, why do you think you were incorrect? According to Table C in this scorecard, what resources should be used and what important assessments should be completed before administering the medication(s)? Did you use these resources and perform these assessments correctly?
- Print a copy of the Medication Scorecard for your instructor to evaluate.

 4. How does the nurse evaluate pain or discomfort in an infant Carrie Richards' age? (*Hint:* See the Pain Intensity section in Chapter 7 of your textbook.)

- Click on **Return to Menu** and then **Restart the Program**.
- Sign in again to work with Carrie Richards (Room 303) during Period of Care 3.
- Click on **Go to Nurses' Station** and then on **303** at the bottom of the screen.
- Click on **Patient Care** and then on **Nurse-Client Interactions**.
- Select and view the video titled **1500: Teaching—Oral Medication**. (*Note:* Check the virtual clock to see whether enough time has elapsed. You can use the fast-forward feature to advance the time by 2-minute intervals if the video is not yet available. Then click again on **Patient Care** and **Nurse-Client Interactions** to refresh the screen.)

5. How does the nurse teach Carrie Richards' mother oral medication administration?

6. What statement(s) does Carrie Richards' mother make about her daughter's eating habits in the last few days prior to admission?

7. What interrelated factors should the nurse consider when an infant has a compromising respiratory illness such as RSV/bronchiolitis and the infant's food intake is decreased?

8. What are the implications of these findings for an infant in relation to hydration status and present illness? (*Hint:* See Water Balance in Infants in Chapter 28 of your textbook.)

9. What concerns does Carrie Richards' mother express about her daughter's nutritional status?

10. How does the nurse address the mother's concerns about Carrie Richards' nutritional status?

LESSON 22

Nutritional Assessment and Discharge Planning

 Reading Assignment: Health Promotion of the Infant and Family (Chapter 12)
Health Problems During Infancy (Chapter 13)
Family-Centered Care of the Child During Illness and
Hospitalization (Chapter 26)

Patient: Carrie Richards, Room 303

Objectives:

1. Assess the nutritional status of the infant with suspected failure to thrive (growth failure).
2. Describe nursing care of the infant with failure to thrive, including family interventions for home care and management.

Exercise 1

 Virtual Hospital Activity

🕐 20 minutes

- Sign in to work at Pacific View Regional Hospital for Period of Care 1. (*Note:* If you are already in the virtual hospital from a previous exercise, click on **Leave the Floor** and then **Restart the Program** to get to the sign-in window.)
- From the Patient List, select Carrie Richards (Room 303).
- Click on **Get Report** and review.
- Click on **Go to Nurses' Station**.
- Click on **Chart** and then on **303**.
- Click on and review the **Emergency Department** record for Carrie Richards.
- Click on and review the **History and Physical**.
- Click on and review the **Nursing Admission** and the **Physician's Orders** for Tuesday 1700 and 2300.

1. What is Carrie Richards' weight on admission to the Emergency Department?

2. What observations are made in the Emergency Department regarding Carrie Richards' body size?

3. What additional observations are made by the staff that address Carrie Richards' overall nutritional status?

4. What is Carrie Richards' secondary medical diagnosis in the Emergency Department?

5. What is the rationale for weighing Carrie Richards again on Wednesday morning at 0755?

6. Review the CDC growth chart on the next page. Based on this chart, Carrie Richards is at the

   _____ percentile for weight-for-age and at the _____ percentile for length-for-age at 3½ months.

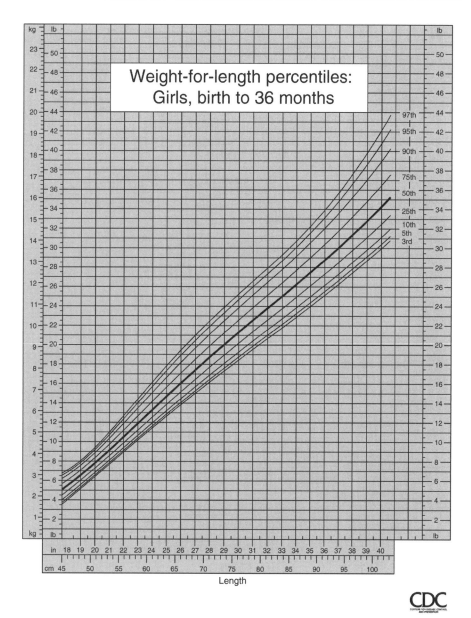

Length

CDC

7. What is the significance of these findings for an infant her age?

➤ • Once again, review Carrie Richards' **History and Physical** and **Nursing Admission** in the chart.

8. In the dietary history there is significant information regarding Carrie Richards' feedings. What does the mother say she has been feeding her daughter? (Include amounts and frequency as applicable.)

 9. What is the significance of this information? (*Hint:* See Nutrition, The First 6 Months, in Chapter 12 in your textbook.)

10. What is the rationale for the addition of rice cereal to a nighttime bottle?

11. Is the practice of placing an infant to sleep with a nighttime bottle recommended? Why?

→ • Click on **Return to Nurses' Station**.
- Click on **303** at the bottom of the screen to go to Carrie Richards' room.
- Click on **Patient Care** and then on **Nurse-Client Interactions**.
- Select and view the video titled **0800: Assessment—Fact Finding**. (*Note:* Check the virtual clock to see whether enough time has elapsed. You can use the fast-forward feature to advance the time by 2-minute intervals if the video is not yet available. Then click again on **Patient Care** and **Nurse-Client Interactions** to refresh the screen.)

12. What assessment does the nurse tell Carrie Richards' mother she will make to assess the child's ability to tolerate feedings in relation to her condition?

13. What additional observations might the nurse make at the time of feeding?

 14. How is the diagnosis of failure to thrive (FTT) established? (*Hint:* See Growth Failure: Diagnostic Evaluation, in Chapter 13 of your textbook.)

Exercise 2

 Virtual Hospital Activity

 15 minutes

- Sign in to work at Pacific View Regional Hospital for Period of Care 2. (*Note:* If you are already in the virtual hospital from a previous exercise, click on **Leave the Floor** and then **Restart the Program** to get to the sign-in window.)
- From the Patient List, select Carrie Richards (Room 303).
- Click on **Go to Nurses' Station**.
- Click on **303** at the bottom of the screen to go to Carrie Richards' room.
- Click on **Patient Care** and then on **Nurse-Client Interactions**.
- Select and view the video titled **1115: Nutritional Assessment**. (*Note:* Check the virtual clock to see whether enough time has elapsed. You can use the fast-forward feature to advance the time by 2-minute intervals if the video is not yet available. Then click again on **Patient Care** and **Nurse-Client Interactions** to refresh the screen.)

1. What does the dietitian report about Carrie Richards' growth failure?

2. During the video, what additional information is discovered about how Carrie Richards is fed that has a significant impact on the number of calories she has been receiving?

3. Based on Carrie Richards' dietary history, which of the following pathophysiologic categories is the most appropriate etiology for her failure to thrive (growth failure)?
   a. Inadequate absorption
   b. Increased metabolism
   c. Defective utilization
   d. Inadequate caloric intake

4. How might the nurse assess the report that Carrie Richards spits up frequently after feedings?

- Click on **Leave the Floor** and then **Restart the Program**.
- Sign in for Period of Care 3 and select Carrie Richards (Room 303).
- Click on **Go to Nurses' Station**.
- Click on **Chart** and then on **303**.
- Click on **Consultations**.
- In the Dietary Consult, review the dietitian's plan for Carrie Richards to achieve catch-up growth in the next few weeks.
- Now click on **Nurse's Notes** and review the notes for Wednesday at 1240, 1425, and 1500.

5. Briefly summarize Carrie Richards' feeding pattern since the acute phase of respiratory distress has resolved and her breathing has improved.

6. Based on Carrie Richards' age and nutritional status, are there any supplements that she should receive? Identify the type as well as the dose of one vitamin supplement that she should start receiving immediately. (*Hint:* See Vitamin Disturbances in Chapter 13 of the textbook.)

7. Write two measurable outcomes for weight gain and caloric (formula) intake for Carrie Richards for the next few days. How will these outcomes be measured?

8. Some interventions have been addressed in regard to Carrie Richards' growth failure. Identify additional nursing interventions that would be appropriate to implement in the hospital setting to help the mother care for her daughter.

Exercise 3

Virtual Hospital Activity

10 minutes

- Sign in to work at Pacific View Regional Hospital for Period of Care 3. (*Note:* If you are already in the virtual hospital from a previous exercise, click on **Leave the Floor** and then **Restart the Program** to get to the sign-in window.)
- From the Patient List, select Carrie Richards (Room 303).
- Click on **Go to Nurses' Station**.
- Click on **Chart** and then on **303**.
- Click on **Consultations** and review the Social Service Consult at 1430 on Wednesday.
- While in the chart, also review the **Nursing Admission** and the **History and Physical**.

1. Describe Carrie Richards' mother's family situation, marital status, sources of economic support, and any other factors that may influence her ability to care for herself and her daughter.

2. Devise a plan for postdischarge follow-up for Carrie Richards and her mother. Consider the mother's lack of transportation, the need for close medical follow-up to assess Carrie Richards' progress over the next few weeks, and limited family resources. Set up the plan for Carrie Richards' Thursday morning discharge and evaluate the feasibility of the plan, assuming that her respiratory status continues to improve as it has since admission Tuesday evening.

23

Emergent Care of the Child with Diabetic Ketoacidosis

 Reading Assignment: Health Promotion of the School-Age Child and Family
(Chapter 17)
Family-Centered Care of the Child During Illness and
Hospitalization (Chapter 26)
Conditions That Produce Fluid and Electrolyte Imbalance
(Chapter 29)
The Child with Endocrine Dysfunction (Chapter 38)

Patient: George Gonzalez, Room 301

Objectives:

1. Recognize the clinical manifestations of diabetic ketoacidosis in a child with type 1 diabetes mellitus.
2. Describe the pathophysiology of diabetic ketoacidosis in a child with type 1 diabetes mellitus.
3. Participate in the nursing care of a child with diabetic ketoacidosis.

Exercise 1

 Virtual Hospital Activity

30 minutes

- Sign in to work at Pacific View Regional Hospital for Period of Care 1. (*Note:* If you are already in the virtual hospital from a previous exercise, click on **Leave the Floor** and then **Restart the Program** to get to the sign-in window.)
- From the Patient List, select George Gonzalez (Room 301).
- Click on **Go to Nurses' Station**.
- Click on **Chart** and then on **301**.
- Click on and review the **Emergency Department** record.

1. What were George Gonzalez's primary and secondary medical diagnoses on admission to the Emergency Department?

2. List five clinical manifestations of diabetic ketoacidosis (DKA).

3. What is the significance of vomiting in a child who has DKA?

4. List altered neurologic signs the nurse should be alert for in a child with DKA.

→ • Click on **Laboratory Reports** and review the initial lab work drawn in the Emergency Department at 1730 on Tuesday.

5. What was George's blood glucose on admission?

6. Briefly explain how an elevated blood glucose level (such as George Gonzalez's) results in dehydration.

7. List the normal blood glucose values for a child George Gonzalez's age. (*Hint:* See Appendix C in your textbook.)

8. Complete the table below with George Gonzalez's lab values and the normal parameters.

Lab Values	George Gonzalez's Values	Normal Values
Sodium (serum)		
Potassium (serum)		
BUN		
Creatinine		
CO_2		
Urine ketones		
Urine glucose		
Urine specific gravity		
Arterial pH		
$PaCO_2$		
PaO_2		
WBC		
Hgb		
Hct		
Platelets		
RBC		

9. Identify the initial intervention performed in the Emergency Department to rehydrate George Gonzalez.

10. Prioritize the following nursing interventions in George Gonzalez's situation by numbering from 1 to 6 (with 1 being the most important intervention and 6 being the least important).

_____ Monitoring for signs/symptoms of potassium imbalance

_____ Monitoring George Gonzalez's glucose level

_____ Monitoring George Gonzalez's neurologic signs

_____ Beginning an infusion of 20 mL/kg isotonic IV solution

_____ Administering 20 units of regular insulin

_____ Placing George Gonzalez on a cardiorespiratory monitor

11. What nursing observations are particularly important for a child with DKA who is receiving IV fluids? (*Hint:* See Diabetes Mellitus: Fluid and Electrolyte Therapy in Chapter 38 of your textbook.)

12. What is the significance of monitoring cardiac function in a child with DKA?

→ • Click on **Physician's Orders** and review the orders for George Gonzalez in the Emergency Department at 1730.

13. What medication is ordered?

To answer the following questions, refer to the Diabetes Mellitus: Therapeutic Management section in Chapter 38 of your textbook.

14. What is the preferred method for administering insulin to a patient with DKA?

15. How was George Gonzalez's insulin administered in the Emergency Department at 1730?

16. What is the significance of admitting a child with DKA to an intensive care unit?

17. What are Kussmaul respirations?

18. What is the significance of Kussmaul respirations in ketoacidosis?

19. Which electrolyte should be monitored carefully in the child with DKA once hydration and insulin administration have been initiated?

20. Before administering the intravenous electrolyte identified in the previous question, it is

   extremely important to ascertain adequate _____ _____ and

   monitor _____ _____ _____.

Care of the Hospitalized Child with Type 1 Diabetes Mellitus

/OTO **Reading Assignment:** The Child with Endocrine Dysfunction (Chapter 38)

Patient: George Gonzalez, Room 301

Objectives:

1. Identify significant diagnostic laboratory tests in the management of type 1 diabetes mellitus.
2. Differentiate between the types of insulin used in the child with type 1 diabetes mellitus.
3. Participate in the care of a child with type 1 diabetes mellitus.

Exercise 1

 Virtual Hospital Activity

 45 minutes

- Sign in to work at Pacific View Regional Hospital for Period of Care 1. (*Note:* If you are already in the virtual hospital from a previous exercise, click on **Leave the Floor** and then **Restart the Program** to get to the sign-in window.)
- From the Patient List, select George Gonzalez (Room 301).
- Click on **Go to Nurses' Station**.
- Click on **Chart** and then on **301** for George Gonzalez's record.
- Review the **History and Physical** and **Nursing Admission** sections of the chart.

1. List the three Ps that are cardinal signs associated with type 1 diabetes mellitus. Briefly explain the significance of each term. Which of these signs did George Gonzalez demonstrate prior to his admission?

2. In the table below list some of the main differences between type 1 and type 2 diabetes mellitus.

Characteristics	Type 1	Type 2
Type of onset		
Sex ratio		
Presenting symptoms		
Nutritional status		
Serum insulin (natural)		
Therapy		
Insulin		
Oral agents		
Diet only		
Chronic complications		
Ketoacidosis		

3. The signs and symptoms of diabetes mellitus may mimic those of other illnesses and may be overlooked. What are some of the illnesses with similar signs and symptoms that may cause one to overlook diabetes mellitus?

→ • Click on **Emergency Department** and review the physician notes.

4. What was George Gonzalez's HgbA1C (glycosylated hemoglobin) on admission to the Emergency Department?

5. What is the significance of George Gonzalez's HgbA1C results in relation to his blood glucose management over the previous 2 to 3 months?

• Click on **Return to Nurses' Station** and then on **301** at the bottom of the screen.
- Click on **Patient Care** and then on **Nurse-Client Interactions**.
- Select and view the video titled **0730: Supervision—Glucose Testing**. (*Note:* Check the virtual clock to see whether enough time has elapsed. You can use the fast-forward feature to advance the time by 2-minute intervals if the video is not yet available. Then click again on **Patient Care** and **Nurse-Client Interactions** to refresh the screen.)

6. What should be the target HgbA1C for George Gonzalez?

7. In this video interaction George Gonzalez makes a statement about how he has managed his diabetes in the past. What does he say about his daily monitoring of glucose and administration of insulin before going to school?

8. What skill does the nurse ask George Gonzalez to perform during this interaction?

9. What is the significance of the nurse observing George Gonzalez check his glucose instead of her checking it for him?

10. What was George Gonzalez's fingerstick blood glucose in the video at 0730?

→ • Click on **Chart** and then on **301**.

• Click on **Physician's Orders** and review the orders written at 2200 on Tuesday.

• Click on **Return to Room 301**.

• Now click on **MAR** and review George Gonzalez's MAR for Wednesday morning.

11. What intervention should occur once George Gonzalez has checked his prebreakfast blood glucose level?

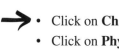 12. Given George Gonzalez's age and developmental level, do you think it is a reasonable expectation for him to be able to test his own glucose at home? (*Hint:* See the section on Diabetes Mellitus: Child and Family Support in Chapter 38 in your textbook.)

13. In addition to monitoring his glucose levels, what additional skill should George Gonzalez be expected to perform in relation to diabetic management?

14. List the doses and types of insulin George Gonzalez is to administer before his breakfast.

15. What is the rationale for using both types of insulin throughout the day?

16. Briefly describe how you would draw up the following: Lispro 6 units and NPH 12 units. Be specific about the order in which you would complete these steps. (*Remember:* Clear insulin, then cloudy insulin.)

Insulin is now available in a number of premixed forms that make administration easier. These forms include the insulin pump and insulin pen. The insulin pump and pen may not be available to all children because of dose and skill level. George Gonzalez may be a candidate for administering insulin with an insulin pen.

17. Briefly describe the advantages of an insulin pen for a person of George Gonzalez's age.

18. Do you believe that George Gonzalez would be a good candidate for an insulin pump at this time? State your rationale.

19. Match each type of insulin below with its corresponding characteristics. (*Hint:* Each insulin type may have more than one matching characteristic.)

Insulin Type	Characteristic
_____ Humalog (lispro H) NovoLog (aspart)	a. Short-acting insulin
	b. Intermediate-acting insulin
_____ NPH or Lente	
	c. Long-acting insulin
_____ Regular	
	d. Injected 15 minutes before meals
_____ UltraLente	

• Click on **Return to Room 301**.
 • Click on **Patient Care** and then on **Nurse-Client Interactions**.
 • Select and view the video titled **0745: Self-Administering Insulin**. (*Note:* Check the virtual clock to see whether enough time has elapsed. You can use the fast-forward feature to advance the time by 2-minute intervals if the video is not yet available. Then click again on **Patient Care** and **Nurse-Client Interactions** to refresh the screen.)

20. In the video, what specific task does the nurse ask George Gonzalez to perform?

21. In this video interaction, how does the nurse evaluate George Gonzalez's understanding of his diabetes?

22. Based on your observation of George Gonzalez's actions in this video and his responses to the nurse about his condition, what conclusions would you draw about George Gonzalez's knowledge regarding diabetes and his subsequent ability to perform glucose monitoring and insulin injection?

23. In this video interaction, George Gonzalez makes a statement that is a key factor in differentiating between the management of type 1 and type 2 diabetes in reference to the need for insulin. What is this statement?

Diabetes Care and Self-Management

 Reading Assignment: Perspectives of Pediatric Nursing (Chapter 1)
Health Promotion of the School-Age Child and Family
(Chapter 17)
Family-Centered Care of the Child with Chronic Illness or
Disability (Chapter 22)
The Child with Endocrine Dysfunction (Chapter 38)

Patient: George Gonzalez, Room 301

Objectives:

1. Describe the significance of glucose monitoring, diet, and exercise in the management of the child with type 1 diabetes mellitus.
2. Discuss the impact of a chronic illness on the preadolescent child and family.

Exercise 1

 Virtual Hospital Activity

55 minutes

- Sign in to work at Pacific View Regional Hospital for Period of Care 2. (*Note:* If you are already in the virtual hospital from a previous exercise, click on **Leave the Floor** and then **Restart the Program** to get to the sign-in window.)
- From the Patient List, select George Gonzalez (Room 301).
- Click on **Go to Nurses' Station**.
- Click on **Chart** and then **301**.
- Click on and review the **Nurses' Notes** and **Physician's Notes**.
- Click on **Return to Nurses' Station** and then **301** at the bottom of the screen to go to George Gonzalez's room.
- Click on **Patient Care** and then on **Nurse-Client Interactions**.
- Select and view the videos titled **1115: Teaching—Disease Process** and **1130: Teaching—Managing Symptoms**. (*Note:* Check the virtual clock to see whether enough time has elapsed. You can use the fast-forward feature to advance the time by 2-minute intervals if the video is not yet available. Then click again on **Patient Care** and **Nurse-Client Interactions** to refresh the screen.)

1. What does George Gonzalez's mother say about his diabetes management?

2. What does George Gonzalez's mother tell the nurse about recognizing his need for insulin?

3. The nurse talks with George Gonzalez's mother about signs indicating that her son may need insulin. What are the signs of hyperglycemia in a child George Gonzalez's age?

4. During these two video interactions, what evaluation is the nurse making regarding George Gonzalez's knowledge of diabetes management?

5. What does George Gonzalez tell the nurse about the signs of hypoglycemia and what he should do if he feels that he is hypoglycemic?

➔ • *Note:* To answer the following two questions, you may need to return to the Nurse-Client Interactions in Period of Care 1 and view the nurse's interactions with George Gonzalez and his mother. (If you need help changing periods of care, see page 16 in the **Getting Started** section of this workbook.)

6. Briefly summarize your impressions regarding the following issues.

   a. George Gonzalez's previous management of diabetes in relation to glucose monitoring and insulin administration

   b. George Gonzalez's mother's knowledge about the importance of daily diabetes management

7. Briefly summarize the main teaching points the nurse has covered up to this point with George Gonzalez and his mother regarding diabetes management.

8. What could the nurse emphasize with George Gonzalez and his mother about diabetes management to help prevent uncontrolled blood glucose and prevent further hospitalizations?

- Click on **Leave the Floor** and then on **Restart the Program**.
- Sign in for Period of Care 3 and select George Gonzalez (Room 301).
- Click on **Go to Nurses' Station**.
- Click on **Chart** and then on **301**.
- Review the **History and Physical** and the **Nursing Admission**.
- Next, click on **Consultations** and review the Psychiatric Consult.

9. According to the History and Physical, George Gonzalez has been hospitalized for problems with diabetes. What specific problems has he had with diabetes management in the last 4 months?

10. List two nursing diagnoses for George Gonzalez based on what you have learned from his chart and the nurse-client interactions.

11. Briefly describe George Gonzalez's family situation (parents, siblings, primary care provider).

12. There are insights to George Gonzalez's previous diabetes management patterns found in the Nursing Admission, History and Physical, and Psychiatric Consult in the chart. List four factors that have contributed to George Gonzalez's noncompliance with the diabetes regimen in the last 4 months.

13. What involvement is expected of George Gonzalez's family, given his age and developmental stage? (*Hint:* See the Diabetes Mellitus: Child and Family Support section in Chapter 38 of your textbook.)

14. George Gonzalez has had diabetes for 4 years. Briefly describe the effect of a chronic illness such as diabetes on a preadolescent and his family. (*Hint:* To learn more about the impact of illness or disability on the preadolescent, see Chapters 17 and 22 in your textbook.)

 15. Define the concept of family-centered care within the context of George Gonzalez's family. (*Hint:* See Chapter 1 of your textbook.)

Exercise 2

 Virtual Hospital Activity

 20 minutes

- Sign in to work at Pacific View Regional Hospital for Period of Care 3. (*Note:* If you are already in the virtual hospital from a previous exercise, click on **Leave the Floor** and then **Restart the Program** to get to the sign-in window.)
- From the Patient List, select George Gonzalez (Room 301).
- Click on **Go to Nurses' Station**.
- Click on **Chart** and then on **301** for George Gonzalez's record.
- Click on **Consultations** and review the Nutrition Consult.
- Click on **Return to Nurses' Station**.
- Click on **301** to go to George Gonzalez's room.
- Inside his room, click on **Patient Care** and then on **Nurse-Client Interactions**.
- Select and view the video titled **1500: Teaching—Diabetic Diet**. (*Note:* Check the virtual clock to see whether enough time has elapsed. You can use the fast-forward feature to advance the time by 2-minute intervals if the video is not yet available. Then click again on **Patient Care** and **Nurse-Client Interactions** to refresh the screen.)

1. What is George Gonzalez's recommended dietary intake?

2. What does the nurse discuss with George Gonzalez in regard to his food intake?

3. What has been George Gonzalez's pattern of eating in the last several months?

4. Describe the relationship of food intake to insulin injections in a child with type 1 diabetes mellitus.

5. How does carbohydrate (CHO) counting give more flexibility in making food choices and administering insulin in children with type 1 diabetes mellitus?

→ • Click on **Patient Care** and then on **Nurse-Client Interactions**.
  • Select and view the video titled **1535: Teaching—Effects of Exercise**. (*Note:* Check the virtual clock to see whether enough time has elapsed. You can use the fast-forward feature to advance the time by 2-minute intervals if the video is not yet available. Then click again on **Patient Care** and **Nurse-Client Interactions** to refresh the screen.)

6. What activity does George Gonzalez say he really likes?

7. Why is exercise an important part of the management of type 1 diabetes?

8. Identify important teaching in the following areas that the nurse should discuss with George Gonzalez in relation to diabetes management and exercise:

a. Glucose monitoring

b. Carbohydrate intake

c. When not to exercise

d. Signs of activity intolerance

9. What specific intervention does George Gonzalez promise to get involved in following discharge that is aimed at helping him manage his diabetes effectively?

10. List additional options that the health care team could discuss with George Gonzalez and his mother to assist in managing his diabetes effectively.